W0254595

Pestilence and Headcolds

This work is a partial representation of *Pestilence and Headcolds* by Sherry Fields, a multimedia work of scholarship published in the Gutenberg-e online history series. As such, this print edition does not include the images, maps or the index contained in the online edition. The Gutenberg-e series is part of our commitment to create new kinds of scholarly and educational publications through new media technologies. Our mission is to make these works as innovative, efficient, and cost-effective as possible. We encourage reviewers and readers to also consult the complete work online at the free access site: http://www.gutenberg-e.org/ or through ACLS Humanities E-Book (HEB) at: http://www.humanitiesebook.org/series_GUTE.html

The online version of this work contains all the printed text here, in addition to digital images, artwork, audio, video, and hyperlinks that allow the reader to experience the full meaning of this scholarly work. The organizing structure, content, and design of the online work was created by the author in collaboration with a team of editors, web developers, and designers in order to give the richest meaning to the historical narrative and argument. The intellectual content of this work is designed to be read and evaluated in its electronic form. This text is not a substitute for or facsimile of the online version of this work.

Pestilence and Headcolds

Encountering Illness in Colonial Mexico

Sherry Fields

www.gutenberg-e.org

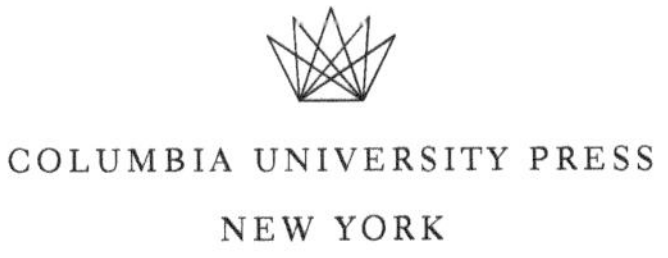

COLUMBIA UNIVERSITY PRESS

NEW YORK

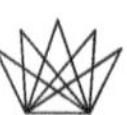

Columbia University Press
Publishers Since 1893
New York Chichester, West Sussex

Library of Congress Cataloging-in-Publication Data

Fields, Sherry Lee.
Pestilence and headcolds : encountering illness in colonial Mexico / Sherry Fields.
p. ; cm.
Originally presented as the author's dissertation (Ph.D.)—University of California, Davis, 2003.
Includes bibliographical references.
ISBN 978-0-231-14240-3 (cloth : alk. paper)
1. Medicine—Mexico—History. 2. Imperialism—Health aspects—Mexico—History. 3. Social medicine—Mexico—History. I. Title.
[DNLM: 1. Sociology, Medical—history—Mexico. 2. Attitude to Health—ethnology—Mexico. 3. Colonialism—history—Mexico. 4. Cultural Diversity—Mexico. 5. History, Modern 1601—Mexico. 6. Religion and Medicine—Mexico. WA 11 DM4 F463p 2008]
R465.F54 2008
362.10972—dc22
2008040360
www.gutenberg-e.org

Columbia University Press books are printed on permanent and durable acid-free paper. This book is printed on paper with recycled content. Printed in the United States of America.

c 10 9 8 7 6 5 4 3 2 1

CONTENTS

ACKNOWLEDGMENTS

Like many first monographs, this book began its life as a PhD dissertation. The road to that dissertation was a very long one—a story I will not bore the reader with here—but I would like to gratefully acknowledge the help I received along the way. Academics normally cite the contributions of family members at the end of their acknowledgments but I must break tradition here. No one deserves my gratitude more than my husband Daniel Fields. His encouragement, sense of pride in my work, and most importantly, unfailing humor kept me moving forward on many difficult days. The content of this book was also greatly enhanced by the many discussions we had about medicine on our evening walks; it was so handy having my own in-house medical resource! Our daughter Rachel—who, growing up, probably thought at one point that all mommies were writing dissertations—added a much-needed balance to my perspective by continually drawing me away from the computer and back to real life.

Almost all my academic training has taken place at UC Davis and I have had many excellent teachers and mentors there throughout the years. Particular thanks go to my dissertation committee members, Arnie Bauer, Chuck Walker, and Andrés Reséndez, for their kind comments and helpful suggestions regarding my work. Arnie, especially, has been an important inspiration in my intellectual journey. My fascination with the history of everyday life was fired by our many discussions, over cappuccinos, about the material culture of life long ago.

My stint in graduate school, particularly the dissertation-writing period, was also brightened considerably by the steadfast optimism of my comrade-in-arms Rosamaria Tanghetti.

I am indebted as well to those individuals who graciously assisted me in countless ways, large and small, with this research. It was Edith Boorstein Couturier who first told me, via an email, about the letters of the Condesa de Miravalle that are housed in the Archivo Manuel Romero de Terreros in Pachuca, Mexico. Belem Oviedo, the director of that archive, made my week-long stay there a productive one. Both Robert McCaa and Paula DeVos generously shared primary sources from their own work. Max and Rosa Shein provided me with useful connections in Mexico City in addition to serving me a lovely lunch. I am also particularly grateful to those individuals and institutions in Mexico that have allowed me to reproduce images from their private collections in this work. Thanks to UC Mexus for the funding, in the form of a Dissertation Research Grant, that launched this project. And lastly, my gratitude goes to the talented people at the Electronic Publishing Initiative at Columbia (EPIC) for transforming my work into its present form as an e-book.

INTRODUCTION

In the summer of 1787, the priest Nicolas Calvo lay suffering in his bed from a serious illness described simply as "malignant dysentery." We know this from the ex-voto he had commissioned to honor the Virgin of Loreto, to whom he attributed his miraculous recovery. His ex-voto opens for us a window onto a part of daily life rarely visited by historians of colonial Spanish America. This is the world of the sick-room, both a physical space abounding with strange tonics and brews, bleedings and leeches, curanderas and barber-surgeons, and saints and virgins, as well as a cultural space complete with its own structures of meaning. This particular ex-voto is especially revealing of the comfortable relationship between divine and rational medicine, two seemingly opposed systems of thought, which, in the disease-laden milieu of eighteenth-century Mexico, tended to complement each other. It shows that even men of religion such as Nicolas Calvo did not entirely trust their health to God. An impressive group of *faculativos* has been called in to assist him, their erudition and status displayed in their clothing, especially in the long cape traditionally worn by the university educated physician, and in the potion bottles and writing instruments pictured on the table beside them. Ultimately, divine medicine wins the day, as it does in all ex-votos, but in this one the earthly practitioners are openly in awe of the Virgin's healing powers (at least according to the ex-voto's creator), admitting great admiration for such a quick recovery under such hopeless circumstances.

But what intrigues the modern viewer most is not so much this friendly competition between divine and rational medicine, but the tiny bit of detail given about the priest's physical condition: "gravely ill from malignant dysentery . . . "some of the tissue of the last intestine had separated," a sign the physicians seem to interpret as certain death. This fascinating fragment of information hints at systems of thought about the body that would be hard to decipher for those of us that use scientific medicine as a way to conceptualize our own bodily functions. My goal in this book is to explore this world of thought through the prism of the sick-room.

A great deal of human suffering caused by illness has marked the history of Mexico through the millennia. Although much of this suffering has been inflicted on great multitudes of people in the form of epidemics, most of it has been the private, and unrecorded, suffering of individuals throughout daily life. Like caprices of nature, illness was arbitrary and inescapable, and people of every age group and social rank moved through life surrounded by its troubling images. Everyone could expect to be assailed, from early childhood on, by a sequence of diseases and disorders, some of them agonizingly painful, and many of them fatal. That morbidity and mortality were high in Mexico's past is supported by a variety of sources. The bioarchaeological record shows that precontact Mexicans were not as healthy as once thought, revealing instead a population that suffered from frequent infection and malnutrition. Both the Mesoamerican and Christian pantheon of gods and saints, mirrors of contemporary anxieties, were created to appeal for divine succor from a vast assortment of afflictions. And so much of the writing of the postconquest era—religious texts, *relaciones*, natural histories, as well as personal letters—reveals an obsession with illness.

One reason death and illness loomed so large in people's minds was that Old World epidemic diseases found very receptive hosts for their pathogens in the virgin-soil populations of the New World. Demographic historians and epidemiologists have focused a great deal of attention on these epidemic diseases, understandably so in view of the tremendous mortality and social dislocation they caused. But an emphasis on epidemics alone distorts our perception of the illnesses that people of the past suffered from in more ordinary times. Other diseases, although not carrying the dramatic impact of severe pestilence, were just as significant in the daily lives of individuals. Perhaps even more interesting for the historian and relevant to the people she studies were the illnesses that did not kill. For every fatal disease, dozens merely disabled, caused pain and discomfort, and disrupted daily lives. People suffered from, and lived with, a multitude of ailments and disorders that today are easily corrected or cured. Maladies of the gastrointestinal track, respiratory problems, eye diseases, dental caries and abscesses, internal parasites, constipation, hemorrhoids, kidney stones, and every sort of skin disease imaginable were all common complaints. Many women, in addition, endured painful gynecological problems caused by multiple and difficult childbirth. And exceptionally large numbers of the physically disabled, blind, and deaf—victims of congenital disorders, dietary deficiencies, infectious disease, and frequent accidents—constituted a common feature of the social landscape.

Why was sickness so ubiquitous? Clearly, the inadequacies of medicine before the nineteenth century contributed to the high rates of illness. Doctors and other caregivers did not fully understand the concept of contagion and had no knowledge of sepsis, immunization, or antibiotics. Far more important, however, were the living conditions of the time. Throughout Mexico's history, the extremely unequal distribution of wealth left most of the population with insufficient access to the basic necessities of housing, clothing, and food. Periodic famine and chronic malnutrition provided a perfect environment for the diffusion of disease, as did the deficiencies of collective and personal hygiene. Those living in urban settings were especially susceptible to falling ill. Water supplies were often contaminated by human and animal wastes, and the accumulation of garbage created an ideal situation for disease-carrying rodents. Such conditions allowed a whole host of human parasites to thrive—not only rats, fleas, and lice, but a variety of microorganisms and worms as well. Even the wealthy could not escape these problems entirely.[1] Yet despite the ubiquity of disease and medical knowledge that was little advanced, this study will show that colonial Mexicans were anything but passive when it came to personal health.

The medical frameworks people use to make sense of their ailments are deeply rooted in their understandings of the relationship between their own physicality and the material conditions in which they live. Everyday beliefs about health and sickness then become basic features in the culture of everyday life, linked in countless ways to the material existence of ordinary people—the foods and drinks they consume, the clothes they wear, the daily habits of grooming, the streets they walk, the houses they live in. If one of the goals of historical research is to get as close as possible to the textures of everyday life of worlds we have lost, then some appreciation of the beliefs people had about their health is essential, especially because the subjects of our historical gaze lived in an age when death rates from infectious disease were so high and life expectancy was so low.

This book explores the cultures of health and illness that were formed amid the high mortality and morbidity rates during the colonial years of Mexico's history. It is concerned first and foremost with the beliefs lay people had about their health: How did they identify and explain their illnesses? Did diseases primarily come from God? Or were there things in the everyday world that could make people sick? What did people imagine to be happening inside their bodies when something went awry? What kinds of things could people do to stay healthy? Did lifestyle effect one's health, and, if so, how? These are the kind of questions that guide this research.

The examination of the illness experience of people long gone is, of course, a fascinating topic, but it also is a rather imprecise enterprise as well, as an infinite variety of circumstances contribute to shape an individual's experience. To simply contemplate the myriad factors affecting just one person's encounter with disease—for example, his or her personal character, the belief systems of the period, the efficacies of the current medical system, the severity and length of illness, access to medical care, and the level of the individual's material life—would probably be enough to discourage even the most ambitious historian, even if she could uncover enough evidence. Outside of an individual's particular situation, broader political and ideological aspects enter into the picture as well. In the case of Mexico, these are fairly easy to identify but harder to flesh out at ground level. Invading Spaniards in the sixteenth century attempted to impose their worldview on the conquered peoples of Mesoamerica—present-day Mexico, Guatemala, and El Salvador—insisting on European forms of settlement and local government, committing themselves to the spread of Christianity, imposing their own notions of racial identity and class, and changing forever native patterns of exchange and consumption. European ideas about the body—resting heavily on the medical concepts of Hippocrates and Galen—were an important part of this imported worldview. The native population had their own notions about disease and the body, of course, concepts that had evolved throughout the various urban-based cultures of Mesoamerica, which, along with the Andes, was one of only two areas of high civilization in the Americas before the European conquest. Precontact medicine combined sophisticated empirical skills, especially in the fields of obstetrics, wound treatment, and herbal remedies, with elaborate forms of shamanism, a practice that naturally conflicted with Christian ideas and their enforcers. The European conquest and, later, its consolidation and expanding settlement meant that Spanish medicine, as practiced by formally educated and examined practitioners, was the only form of healing to be legally recognized by colonial authorities. But reality on the ground—ridiculously low numbers of "qualified" physicians and surgeons coupled with massive numbers of people needing medical attention—made this impossible. Consequently, a whole host of irregular curers, most of them with some empirical know-how, but many charlatans as well, flourished in the cities, towns, and countryside of New Spain. To approach the illness experience of colonial Mexicans, then, we need to keep in mind that our analytical spectrum incorporates an astonishingly wide range of belief systems and social experience. Such a broadly cast net is unavoidable in an exploratory study such as this one.

Undoubtedly, some readers will find this focus on the ailing bodies of historical actors gloomy, "one long bellyache, a primal scream against the atrocities perpetuated by Nature and by social oppression."[2] Others likely will argue that such a topic is historically insignificant because human beings, at all places and times in their evolution, have suffered from disease and thus to stress this is to say nothing particular about a historical period. But to exclude the experience of the individual, as so much of orthodox medical history has done, seriously depersonalizes illness, reducing it to a black box on a histogram. It also tends to minimize the complexity disease has as a social phenomenon and, by extension, a shaper of history. "Disease," writes one historian,

> Is at once a biological event, a generation-specific repertoire of verbal constructs reflecting medicine's intellectual and institutional history, an occasion of and potential legitimization for public policy, an aspect of social role and individual—intrapsy chic—identity, a sanction for cultural values, and a structuring element in doctor and patient interactions. In some ways disease does not exist until we have agreed that it does, by perceiving, naming, and responding to it.[3]

At its most basic level, illness colors everyday experiences by way of the physical suffering and mental anxiety (brought on, no doubt, by our innate fear of death) it produces in individuals and communities.

The study of health, illness, and medicine in Mexico contains a curious discrepancy between what we know about lay conceptions of medicine in recent times and those in past centuries. Anthropologists in the twentieth century, especially since the 1960s, have produced a plethora of case studies that attempt to map the ethnomedical systems of contemporary Mexican communities.[4] These studies show that many Mexicans continue to filter their observations of the body through conceptual frameworks inherited from their colonial ancestors. Curanderos and other traditional healers still treat illnesses such as evil eye, *susto*, and soul loss through a combination of ritual and herbal remedies, and popular beliefs about the curing powers of saints and local virgins continue to be widespread.[5] Age-old empirical knowledge easily coexists alongside modern medicine. Although caregivers in the home today will utilize aspirin and antibiotics, they are also as likely to incorporate "the principle of opposites" in explaining and treating sickness, thus stipulating that a "hot" remedy be used for a "cold" illness, or vice versa. Foods are thought to have "hot" and "cold" qualities: honey, coffee, and beef (especially from a bull) are hot, whereas turkey, rice, *jícama*, and limes are cold.[6] Both Spanish and Mesoamerican medicine used the Hot-Cold dichotomy in precontact and colonial times to diagnose and treat illnesses, so it is difficult to untangle the origins of these folk practices today.[7] As we will see in this study, however, the humoral medicine that Europeans brought to the New World provided a logical and simple framework on which both indigenous and popular Spanish curing practices could be hung.

Although much has been written about popular medical concepts and practices in twentieth-century Mexico, work on their historical evolution has been less prolific. Scholars have been fascinated, of course, with the extent and demographic consequences of epidemic diseases in Mexico's past, especially those of the sixteenth century, which were catastrophic for the native population.[8] But most of the published historiography focusing on medicine has consisted of biographies of doctors and studies of medical institutions. Some of these studies have documented the founding and administration of several of the many hospitals that were established by religious groups and the Spanish Crown in early years of the colony. Other institutional studies have included work on the Protomedicato, the medical board responsible for overseeing the education and licensing of medical practitioners in Spain and her colonies.[9] Very recent studies include one that skillfully traces the development of pharmaceutical practice from art to science in the seventeenth and eighteenth centuries and a collection of essays on various topics relating to the practice of medicine in New Spain.[10] Precontact medicine has received serious scholarly attention, especially from Alfredo López Austin, whose meticulous study of Nahua concepts of the body was based on his close reading of the Nahuatl language and colonial indigenous sources.[11] And, finally, a couple of excellent studies have begun the process of looking at the everyday world of colonial lay medicine. Both focus on supernatural beliefs and practices and are based on extensive work in the vast collection of inquisitional records, which document the prosecution of curanderos during the three centuries of Spanish rule in Mexico.[12] All of these works form an indispensable background and basis for the present study, as does much of the excellent, and much more extensive, medical historiography done on early modern Europe cited throughout this book.

What kinds of historical sources does one dig through to find out what people of past centuries thought about health and illness? The most fertile documents have been those in which lay people mention their own illness experience firsthand or that of family members. Personal letters are rich with such incidents, although it has been difficult to find many of them for colonial Mexico. For the present study, I have used two collections of letters. Enrique Otte's superb compilation of letters written by Spanish emigrants in the sixteenth century to family and acquaintances in Spain contains fascinating tidbits for the researcher on many subjects, including health. Almost all of the letters mention health, at least in passing, and many describe experiences with illness, accidents, doctors, and the death of loved ones. The other collection consists of the personal correspondence of the Countess of Miravalle, a well-connected but indebted widow, to her son-in-law, Pedro Romero de Terreros, a wealthy mining magnate and the first Conde de Regla.[13] In 1756, the forty-three-year-old Romero de Terreros married the twenty-three-year-old María Antonia, the Condesa's youngest daughter. Ten years and at least nine pregnancies later, María Antonia died, ending the close association between the Condesa and her son-in-law. The letters written by the Condesa during this decade-long correspondence, which are housed in the Archivo Manuel Romero de Terreros in Pachuca, Mexico, contain much commentary about the family's state of health and a great deal of health advice from the Condesa herself.

Sickness and health are also frequently mentioned in contemporary writings such as travelers' accounts, correspondence of religious and political officials, chronicles, newspapers, and especially in the *Relaciones Geográficas*. Sometimes the authors are eyewitnesses to an illness experience, either their own or that of others. Antonio de Ciudad Real, who narrates the journey of Fray Alonoso Ponce, a commissary-general touring Franciscan convents during the 1580s, describes, at times in vivid detail, Ponce's health problems and the efforts of others to relieve him.[14] But mostly these writings yield information about lay health concepts by inference; comments on food and clothing, for instance, or climate and location are very revealing of how preindustrial peoples viewed the relationship between human bodies and the environment, a topic that we cover in depth in this book. In this regard, the *Relaciones Geográficas*, the questionnaire sent out by Philip II to take stock of his American possessions, contains an especially rich layer of information about Spanish etiology, gleaned from comments about such things as indigenous lifestyle, the geography and climate of Indian towns, and native remedies. In addition, *La Gaceta de México*, a newspaper published in the eighteenth century, offers an abundance of information about the health concerns of the day. Its pages are filled with the news of epidemics, announcements about new therapies and medicines, strange deaths, divine cures, and specialized practitioners advertising their skills.

Another source for exploring lay health concepts is the growing body of vernacular books on medicine emerging in sixteenth- and seventeenth-century Mexico. Works written by professionals may seem an unlikely place to look for lay perspectives, but for most of the early modern period the boundaries between professional and lay medical cultures are still so blurred that it is simply anachronistic to imagine them as the discrete realms they are today. Most educated people knew something about medicine, while formally trained physicians and surgeons drew on a widely shared empirical tradition. Several works directed at the layperson—home medical guides, or *recetarios*—were published in the colonial period, their authors citing the lack of doctors and pharmacies as important reasons for producing these books. The surgeon Alonso López de Hinojosos, whose book *Suma y recopilación de cirugia con un arte para sangrar muy útil y provechosa* was published in Mexico City in 1578, wrote this work for: "those that are outside of the city in mines and *estancias,* towns and remote areas, who lack the convenient remedies."[15] Juan de Esteyneffer's *Florilegio medicinal de todas las enfermedades sacado de varios y clásicos autores para bien de los pobres y de los que tiene falta de médicos* was probably one of the most popular, and enduring, medical guides ever published for the layman. The Moravian Esteyneffer came to Mexico in 1697 as a Jesuit missionary and, although not formally trained as a physician, quickly gained fame for his knowledge of medicine. While working in the Jesuit missions of northern Mexico, he wrote the *Florilegio* to assist the missionary effort, which had few formal medical resources at hand. Because the book is so reader-friendly—its chapters are laid out according to type of ailment, arranged in a logical head-to-toe order (thus, headaches come before disorders of the eyes, followed by those of the nose and mouth, moving downward through the body), its recipes easy to follow and make, using "simples," or single-ingredient remedies, and native ingredients whenever possible—it was a great success. After its first appearance in Mexico City in 1712, the *Florilegio* went through at least five other editions, the last of which was published in Mexico in 1887. Anecdotal evidence suggests that a few curanderas still find it useful: during the 1970s an anthropologist studying popular medicine in the Oaxacan backcountry encountered a *zapoteca* who consulted this book almost daily when the pueblo's sick came to her for advice. Her copy was a 1755 edition, lacking cover, title page, and author, and had been handed down through the family's female line for over two hundred years.[16]

I found the colonial *recetarios* fascinating reading for several reasons. For one, they are a superb source for contemporary descriptions of the disorders of the day; within these pages we find lengthy descriptions of *dolor de costado, flaqueza del estomago, dolor de ijada, morbo gálico, obstrucción del hígado, mal de madre, apostemas,* and *tabardillo.* Several of them also provide important information about the causes of diseases, which, according to the authors, are frequently found in the environment and lifestyle choices of patients. Other colonial texts, not necessarily remedy books, but works of general health advice, are also quite revealing about how people conceptualized the linkage between day-to-day life and disease, in addition to being greatly entertaining to read.[17]

And, finally, a word about ex-votos. These small votive paintings, which were (and, in some places, still are) left in shines as gestures of gratitude for divine intervention, visually complement the textual sources used for this study of lay medical cultures in New Spain. Like Nicolas Calvo's, with which I began this Introduction, all ex-votos have one common theme: surviving the calamities of everyday life. Spontaneous and formulaic at the same time, they combine visual representation—the suffering patient in sick-bed, the scene of an accident, the kneeling supplicant—with textual information about the life-threatening incident and the miraculous intervention of a beloved virgin or saint. Although the majority of historical ex-votos housed in museums, sanctuaries, and private collections are from the national period, when the practice spread to the popular classes, I have tried to limit my use of them here to those produced during the colonial years, even though they are less plentiful than the later ones and were generally commissioned by people exclusively from the upper and middle classes. What kind of information can we glean from these images? In a way they are very much like the personal correspondence of the time: individual testimonies, many of them offering up intriguing bits and pieces—like Nicolas Calvos's intestines—that force us to dig deeper elsewhere. But sometimes we get lucky and they contain a richly detailed narration of experience, as do a few of the ones I have used here. They also bring to our story a viewpoint that the medical guides do not; that is, they underscore the essential role that miracle healing played in this colonial world of sickness and suffering, an important phenomenon in an age when the efficacy of rational medicine was woefully inadequate. And, finally, their visual quality somewhat enhances, I think, our link to the subjects of this study; pictures capture pathos in a way that textual evidence does not.

Perhaps it is already evident to the reader that our examination here is essentially an impressionistic one, a preliminary study on which future research can build. With few secondary sources to work from, this initial sketch of colonial Mexican sickness cultures simply seeks to lay a groundwork by exploring a variety of sources that might, or might not, yield promising evidence for other projects such as this one. It is for this reason that findings here are presented with such broad strokes. Nowhere in this dissertation do I address in depth those modes of analysis so dear to the hearts of specialists. Class, gender, and ethnic divisions are, of course, important determinants in how everyday life gets played out, but, at this stage at least, their role in shaping the variety of medical experience in colonial Mexico is not explored in any comprehensive way. I have begun, instead, with a more simplistic analytical approach by looking at, and at times comparing, European and indigenous notions of the body and its disorders. Because most of our knowledge about Mesoamerican culture comes from early colonial sources that focus on the Nahuas, those inhabitants living in the core regions of central Mexico by the fifteenth and sixteenth centuries, general comments about indigenous concepts and practices refer to that cultural group. Likewise, my efforts to understand colonial indigenous approaches to health are based almost entirely here on those views of precontact life that were recorded in the early years of Spanish rule. Another unavoidably vague generalization in this bird's-eye view is periodization. Although my intention here is to paint a broad picture of colonial life, I am well aware that people living in the 1570s had a different outlook and sensibility than their counterparts living in the 1770s. But these are differences that cannot be explored here. Thus, I use the term "colonial" in a very loose way, shamelessly lumping together ideas from the sixteenth century with those of the later years of Spanish rule. One thing did unite the beginning and end of the colonial period, however, and that is the vulnerability people felt toward the relentless roll of disease for which contemporary medicine had very few effective responses.

Although the real task for any study concerned with understanding the experience of illness is to identify the sufferers' patterns of thought and action, one must begin first with the basic circumstances surrounding health. The first two chapters of this book do just that. In Chapter 1, I examine the kinds of diseases and ailments people suffered from in Mexico, beginning with precontact Mesoamerica on the eve of the Spanish Conquest up to roughly the middle of the nineteenth century. In addition to the deadly diseases, which attacked in both epidemic and endemic forms, I look at the disorders people routinely lived with as well. Chapter 2 continues this examination with a look at the medical market place, that is, at the vast assortment of people dispensing medical services, licensed and unlicensed, that competed in an environment where the consumer remained largely in charge of his or her own care. We begin this exploration of healers with a brief look at the great variety of medical specialists that existed in precontact central Mexico. In the following two chapters, which form the core of this study, I explore the notions people had about the origins of their diseases and staying healthy, and by extension, their ideas about how their bodies worked. The illness experience of colonial indigenous peoples is not accessible to us unless we know something about precontact practices and concepts. Chapter 3 therefore looks at Mesoamerican notions of the body, illness, and health, aspects of daily life that were deeply linked to religion in ways Europeans found difficult to understand or tolerate. Chapter 4 looks at these same concepts through a European worldview, specifically through the prism of humoral medicine on which Spanish notions of the body were based. Although European bodies also were subject to the mysterious workings of divine powers, they were far more vulnerable to the physical worlds in which they lived. Environment and lifestyle played critical roles in the health of those colonial inhabitants that lived within a European cultural sphere. In Chapter 5, I conclude this study with a bit more probing into the illness experiences of colonial Mexicans by, first, considering some of the ways health concerns textured daily life and, second, by briefly looking at how Mexican Catholicism shaped the encounter with disease.

NOTES

1. On living conditions in late colonial cities, see Martha Eugenia Rodríguez, *Contaminación e insalubridad en la ciudad de México en el siglo XVIII* (México: Dept. de Historia y Filosofía de la Medicina/ Falcultad de Medicina, UNAM, 2000); Miguel Ángel Cuenya Mateos, *Puebla de los Ángeles en tiempos de una peste colonial: una mirada en torno al matlazahuatl de 1737* (Zamora: El Colegio de Michoacán, Benemérita Universidad Autónoma de Puebla, 1999).

2. Roy Porter, "The Patient's View: Doing Medical History from Below," *Theory and Society*, 14 (1985), p. 182.

3. Charles E. Rosenberg, "Framing Disease: Illness, Society, and History," in *Framing Disease: Studies in Cultural History*, ed. Charles E. Rosenberg and Janet Golden (New Brunswick, NJ: Rutgers University Press, 1992), p. xiii.

4. See George Foster, *Hippocrates' Latin American Legacy: Humoral Medicine in the New World* (Amsterdam: Gordon and Breach Science Publishers, 1992); Isabel Kelly, *Folk Practices in North Mexico: Birth Customs, Folk Medicine, and Spiritualism in the Laguna Zone* (Austin: University of Texas Press, 1965); John L. Gwaltney, *The Thrice Shy: Cultural Accommodation to Blindness and Other Disasters in a Mexican Community* (New York: Columbia University Press, 1970); John M. Ingham, "On Mexican Folk Medicine," *American Anthropologist*, 72:1 (Feb. 1970), 76–87.

5. See Bonnie Bade, "Contemporary Mixtec Medicine: Emotional and Spiritual Approaches to Healing, in *Cloth and Curing: Continuity and Change in Oaxaca*, ed. Grace Johnson and Douglas Sharon (San Diego: San Diego Museum Papers, 1994); Frank Lipp, *The Mixe of Oaxaca: Religion, Ritual, and Healing* (Austin: University of Texas Press, 1991).

6. Foster, p. xv.

7. The debate about the origins of the Hot-Cold dichotomy has engaged anthropologists for at least two decades, but the principle advocates of each side seem to be Alfredo López Austin, who argues for an American origin, and Geoge Foster, who claims these practices are legacies of Spanish humoral medicine. See Alfredo López Austin, *The Human Body and Ideology: Concepts of the Ancient Nahuas*, 2 vols., trans. Thelma Ortiz de Montellano and Bernard Ortiz de Montellano (Salt Lake City: University of Utah Press, 1988), pp. 270–82; and Foster, pp. 147–87.

8. Enrique Florescano and Elsa Malvido, *Ensayos sobre la historia de las epidemias en México*, 2 vols. (México: Instituto Mexicano del Seguro Social, 1982); Alfred W. Crosby Jr., "Conquistador y pestilencia: The First New World Pandemic and the Fall of the Great Indian Empires," *HAHR* 47 (1967), 321–37; Alfred W. Crosby Jr., *The Columbian Exchange: Biological and Cultural Consequences of 1492* (Westport, CT: Greenwood Press, 1972); Robert McCaa, "Spanish and Nahuatl Views on Smallpox and Demographic Catastrophe in Mexico," *Journal of Interdisciplinary History*, XXV:3 (Winter 1995), 397–431; Noble David Cook and W. George Lovell, *Secret Judgements of God: Old World Disease in Colonial Spanish America* (Norman: University of

Okalahoma Press, 1991); Thomas M. Whitmore, *Disease and Death in Early Colonial Mexico: Simulating Amerindian Depopulation* (Boulder, CO: Westview Press, 1992); Shelburne F. Cook and Woodrow Borah, *Essays in Population History,* 3 vols. (Berkeley: University of California Press, 1971–9).

9. Josefina Mureil, *Hospitales de Nueva España,* 2 vols. (México: Publicaciones del Instituto de Historia, 1956); David A. Howard, *The Royal Indian Hospital of Mexico City* (Tempe: Arizona State University, 1980); J. Joaquín Izquierdo, *Raudon, cirujano poblano de 1810: aspectos de la cirugia mexicana de principios del siglo XIX en torno de una vida* (México: Ediciones Cinecia, 1949); Joaquín García Icazbalceta, *Los médicos de México en el siglo XVI* (México: Imprenta de V. Agueros, 1896); Francisco Fernández del Castillo, *La cirugia mexicana en los siglos XVI & XVII* (New York: Squibb & Sons, 1936); Fernando Cortés Martínez, *Historia general de la medicina en México* (México: UNAM, 1984); John Tate Lanning, *The Royal Protomedicato,* (Durham, NC: Duke University Press, 1985); Luz María Hernández Sáenz, *Learning to Heal: The Medcial Profession in Colonial Mexico, 1767–1831* (New York: Peter Lang, 1997).

10. Paula De Vos, "The Art of Pharmacy in Seventeenth- and Eighteenth-Century Mexico," Ph.D. dissertation (University of California, Berkeley, 2001); Enrique Cárdenas de la Peña, ed., *Temas medicos de la Nueva España* (México: Instituto Cultural Domecq, A.C., 1992).

11. López Austin, *The Human Body and Ideology;* see also Alfredo López Austin, "Cosmovición y salud entre los mexicas," in *Historia general de la medicina en México,* Vol. 1, eds. Alfredo López Austin and Carlos Viesca Treviño (México: UNAM, Academia Nacional de Medicina, 1984); Bernard R. Ortiz de Montellano, *Aztec Medicine, Health, and Nutrition* (New Brunswick, NJ: Rutgers University Press, 1994); Carlos Viesca Treviño, "Prevencion y terapeúticas mexicas," and "El médico mexica," in López Austin and Viesca Treviño, eds.; Carlos Viesca Treviño, *Medicina prehispánica de México: El conocimiento médico de los nahuas* (México: Panorama Editorial, 1986).

12. Gonzalo Aguirre Beltran, *Medicina y magia: El proceso de aculturación en la estructura colonial* (México: Instituto Nacional Indigenista, 1963); Neomí Quezada, *Enfermedad y malefación, el curandero en el México colonial* (México: UNAM, 1989).

13. Enrique Otte, *Cartas privadas de emigrantes a Indias, 1540–1616* (México: Fondo de Cultura Económica, 1993); Archivo Manuel Romero de Terreros, *Miravalles,* Pachuca, Mexico.

14. Antonio de Cuidad Real, *Tratado curioso y docto de las grandezas de la Nueva España,* 2 vols., eds., Josefina García Quintana, Victor M. Castillo Farreras (México: UNAM, 1993).

15. Alonso López de Hinojosos, *Suma y recopilación de cirugía con un arte para sangrar muy útil y provechosa* (México: Academia Nacional de Medicina, 1977), p. 77.

16. Juan de Esteyneffer, *Florilegio medicinal de todas las enfermedades sacados de various y clásicos autores para bien de los pobres y de los que tienen falta de médicos,* 2 vols., ed. Ma. del Carmen Anzures y Bolaños (México: Academia Nacional de Medicina, 1978), pp. 20–25, 31.

17. Juan de Cárdenas, *Problemas y secretos maravillosos de las Indias* (Madrid: Alianza Editorial, 1988); Luis Lobera de Avila, *Banquete de nobles caballeros* (Madrid: Reimpresiones Bibliográficas, 1952); Cristobal Mendez, *The Book of Bodily Exercise*, trans. Francisco Guerra, ed. Frederick G. Kilgour (New Haven, CT: Elizabeth Licht, 1960).

1. PESTILENCE AND HEADCOLDS

Was there ever a time in humanity's history that did not include disease? The ancient Greeks mark the beginning of pestilence and other torments of the flesh by the fable of Pandora's box, whereas the Judeo-Christian tradition explains that disease and death became part of the human condition when Eve successfully tempted Adam into tasting the forbidden fruit. Today we know that the diseases of humanity evolved in tandem with its civilizations. Beginning roughly 11,000 years ago, various peoples began the slow process of domesticating animals and plants, ultimately setting the stage for the development of what Jared Diamond has aptly called "guns, germs, and steel." This transition from hunter-gatherers to farmers set off a long chain of events in the evolution of humanity. The cultivation of crops and herd animals allowed for surplus food production, which led to a sedentary lifestyle, a growing population in more densely packed living conditions, and non-food-producing specialists. These specialists, in turn, evolved into roles we now associate with civilized societies: political elites, bureaucrats, priests, artisans, and scribes. Travel, trade, and warfare, all impossible without domesticated animals serving as land transport and carriers of goods, soon followed, intermingling humans as never before. Infectious diseases arose right alongside this sequence of civilizing advancements. Those farmers and herdsmen who were the first to raise large quantities of crops and animals also unintentionally produced large numbers of human predators:

rats, roaches, houseflies, mosquitoes, worms, fungi, and bacteria. The resulting "diseases of civilization"—smallpox, measles, typhus, and the flu—began, researchers now tell us, in the close physical relationship the Old World's peoples had with their herds of cattle, sheep, goats, horses, and pigs. Thus, the real origins of humanity's diseases are found in its greatest achievements.[1]

As everyone now knows, these pathogens eventually played a critical role in the conquests of the New World, whose inhabitants had no immunity to the Old World diseases brought by the conquistadors and early settlers. This virulent and, from the point of view of the sufferers, incomprehensible onslaught of disease marks a decisive moment in Mexico's history. It also forms the most dramatic part of our story about the connections between the quest for health and everyday life in New Spain. But even in times when pestilence was subdued, ordinary illnesses and bodily discomforts were daily preoccupations for all groups of society. With this chapter, we begin our look at the circumstances surrounding health by identifying and describing—in the sufferers' own words whenever possible—the maladies that afflicted Mexicans before the arrival of modern medicine. We begin with Mesoamerica, where recent scholarship has uncovered new clues about the overall health of ancient Mexicans. The rest of this chapter explores the health problems of the inhabitants of New Spain, beginning with the frequent outbreaks of pestilence and other infectious diseases, on through to the more common ailments of everyday life.

ANCIENT MESOAMERICA

In sharp contrast to the images of death and destruction initiated by the European conquest, precontact American populations have often been depicted by popular, and some scholarly, interpretations, in almost utopian terms. Lately, this image of strong, vigorous, and healthy populations living in a pre-Columbian paradise is being challenged by scholars examining the skeletal evidence of early settlements. Recent paleodemographic studies are revealing Mesoamericans as having been more similar to their Old World contemporaries than previously thought. Short, hard lives plagued by poor nutrition and ill health were the rule for most ordinary people. Although the pre-Columbian populations may not have suffered from the waves of epidemics that killed so many people in Old World cities, the evidence shows that physiological stress in the form of infection and undernutrition was common, if not chronic, in many ancient Mesoamerican urban settlements. Calculations of life expectancy point to short lives: at birth, life expectancy was only 15–20 years; if one made it to age 15, he or she could expect to live another 13 to 29 years, in other words, to age 28 through 44 on average. Estimates of infant mortality have been put as high as around 30 percent—40 percent. These figures show two things: that infancy was perhaps the most perilous stage in a person's life; and, this extremely high death rate of infants and children was what kept these growing populations—women averaged 8.8 births in their lifetime—in check.[2]

Most historians agree that the populations of precontact America did not suffer from the "crowd-type" epidemic diseases that afflicted Old World cities, the reasons for which will be discussed later in this chapter. This does not mean, however, that there were no epidemics. Mesoamerican sources mention pestilence as one of the calamities that occurred periodically, usually during a time of prolonged famine. The *Historia chichimeca* tells of a "*catarro pestilencial*" that came during the unusually cold weather of 1454, from which many people died. For the next three years, an unremitting cycle of drought and freezing temperatures brought about a catastrophic situation for the Nahuas, as they endured the twin scourges of hunger and sickness.[3] But information about the health of pre-Colombians is still too meager to even speculate on what diseases would have periodically reached epidemic levels. Their endemic diseases and health problems, however, are being made more visible by the recent work of paleopathologists.[4] Skeletal remains, the primary source of evidence for these scholars, contains a considerable amount of data about the physical lives of people from all periods of Mesoamerican history. Although not as revealing as soft tissue, human bones, nonetheless, record important information about causes of death, the incidence and severity of chronic diseases, traumas from accidents or warfare, and the biomechanical patterns from habitual work. Interpretation of the skeletal record, however, is not perfect, as not all diseases affect bone and some diseases can affect bone in similar ways.[5]

Many scholars have theorized a correlation between the rise of agriculture and the increased incidence of disease in ancient populations. The general notion is that as populations shifted their subsistence from foraging to agriculture their settlement pattern changed from mobility to sedentism. An increasing population density led to sanitation problems, producing ideal conditions for the spread of infectious disease. Large urban populations also entailed increasing social complexity, creating inequalities of wealth and access to basic resources.[6] Temporal trends in precontact Central Mexico, with its long history as the center of Mesoamerican civilization, seem to support this hypothesis. Skeletal evidence shows a general trend of increased incidence of disease as Mesoamerica evolved from the Preclassic period (1600 BC–AD 300)—where the densest settlements were villages, where social and economic differentiation was present but not greatly elaborated, and where subsistence was based on agriculture but supplemented regularly by foraging of wild resources—to the

Classic (AD 300–900) and Postclassic (900–1521) periods. In these latter epochs, more and more people came to live in densely populated cities with poor sanitary conditions, ate a more monotonous diet based on squash, corn, and beans, and experienced much greater social and economic differentiation. This change in the way people lived coincided with a trend toward a decline in the stature of Mesoamericans, from the Preclassic to the Postclassic. Shortening stature may have been an adaptive response to malnutrition, under-nutrition, and chronic infection in childhood.[7] Like preindustrial cities in Europe, Mesoamerican urban settings with dense populations are believed to have had problems with public sanitation and contaminated water supplies, which help explain their high rates of infectious diseases and high mortality. Although cities in central Mexico like Teotihuacan and Tenochtitlan were situated in an arid highland environment, which would have been beneficial in curtailing the threat of some diseases spread by insects, it would have been difficult to prevent contamination of the water supply. This part of North America has a monsoonal rain pattern, where most of its rain falls from the beginning of the month of June through September, while the rest of the year receives trivial quantities of rainfall—too little to refresh nearby reservoirs. Residents of these urban areas would have drawn some of their drinking water from year-round springs, but the reservoirs and lakes surrounding the cities would have also served as a fresh water source. During the dry season, without the rains to wash away much of the human waste and trash, these bodies of waters would have been the source of many parasitic and endemic intestinal infections. The newborns and young children of these settlements would have been especially vulnerable in such an environment because an important cause of neonatal mortality is infection. Infants can become infected with such diseases as conjunctivitis, pneumonia, osteomyetitis, and meningitis, to name a few that were probably present in ancient Mesoamerica. Moreover, the bacteria that cause diarrhea are easily transmitted to babies at birth from an infected birth canal or the hands of birth attendants and parents. These diarrheal infections are the kinds of illnesses that would have run rampant in the urban settings of Mesoamerica, where inadequate disposal of human wastes and a lack of water for cleaning, especially during dry periods, would have created the perfect environment for pernicious viruses.[8]

Mesoamerican skeletons also reveal that a settled way of life was hard on the joints and teeth. One way in which the Old and New Worlds differed was the latter's lack of beasts of burden (except the llama, which carried light loads) and technology which aided in strenuous tasks, such as the wheel or iron tools. Mesoamerica was a society powered largely by human muscle. Human bodies were the principle mechanism for growing food, erecting buildings, and transporting heavy burdens and goods. Hard and repetitive work imposed a severe toll on the bodies of both men and women, especially on the joints required for mobility, manipulation of objects, or bearing loads.[9] Skeletal evidence from the Classic and Postclassic periods tends to show a higher occurrence of degenerative joint disease than populations from earlier times, reflecting the biomechanical stress that common people might have experienced when they shifted from a hamlet-like subsistence economy to an urban one based on trade. The wear and tear on Mesoamerican joints also reflects the division of work along gender lines. Women display significantly more joint disease of the wrists than men, not surprising given that the preparation of maize tortillas, the main source of calories, was a laborious task that had to be preformed twice a day by the women of the family. Men, the carriers of heavy loads, tend to show greater mechanical stress in the neck and lumbar region.[10] Life based on agriculture also took its toll on the teeth of Mesoamericans. Although the dental wear and tear caused by the consumption of foraged foods was reduced over time, dental caries, abscesses, and tooth loss became more pronounced as high-carbohydrate, maize-based diets became the norm.[11]

What kinds of infectious diseases might have afflicted the inhabitants of Mesoamerica? Skeletal evidence for tuberculosis and treponemal infection—forms of syphilis and yaws—have been found throughout the Americas, including Mexico.[12] Whether or not this included venereal syphilis is still one of the most widely debated subjects in medical historiography, and one that I explore later in this chapter. It is likely, however, that some forms of venereal disease existed in Mesoamerica; "putrefaction of the member" is mentioned as a divine punishment for violation of ritual abstinence and medicines to treat male and female genitalia were listed in a native herbal.[13] The most common aliments, however, were probably gastrointestinal and respiratory infections. These would have included things such as bacillary and amoebic dysentery, viral influenza and pneumonia, bacterial pathogens like staphylococcus and streptococcus, salmonella and other food poisoning agents, and various internal parasites. Shelburn Cook found that the Mexican *materia medica* indeed included an abundance of remedies for these types of illnesses. Based on the assumption that "any civilization relying upon an herbalistic rational of medicine inevitably tends to find a preponderance of medicines for those ailments that are both most common and most lethal," he compared Mexican remedies with those of contemporary Europe. His conclusion was that inflammatory and febrile infections were more prevalent in semi-tropical Mexico than in temperate Europe.[14] Unfortunately, as soon as Europeans landed on the coast of Mexico in 1519, the extent and variety of Mesoamerican diseases increased rapidly, and with devastating consequences.

COLONIAL MEXICO

Historians concerned with the story of disease in New Spain have centered their gaze, for the most part, on the horrific epidemics that nearly wiped out the indigenous population in the sixteenth century. Thanks to their work over the last thirty years, we have become more aware of the crucial role infectious diseases played in the conquest and colonization of the New World by Europeans. According to one of the pioneers of this field: "The fatal diseases of the Old World killed more effectively in the New, and the comparatively benign diseases of the Old World turned killer in the New."[15] Scholars have shown comparatively little interest, however, in the endemic and chronic diseases of the day, which surely formed a greater part of everyday experience than the periodic outbreak of pestilence during which "normality" was suspended. One of the central assertions of this study is that the illness experiences of people in the past were very different than our own. Modern medicine has not only made enormous strides against infectious diseases—yesterday's great killers—but has significantly increased life expectancy, reduced our discomfort level from chronic disease and injuries through painkillers and highly technical surgical procedures, and medicalized death to such an extent that the passing of family and friends usually takes place away from our view and immediate experience. In contrast, the ubiquity of illness and, perhaps even more significantly, the likelihood of early death were simply part of the everyday landscape of the past, producing, certainly, a considerable effect on the *mentalité* of the time.[16] Indeed, colonial sources for Mexico show that people were regularly watchful to all sorts of changes in their health and intensely concerned about the consequence of apparently trivial symptoms.

We begin here our look at the broad spectrum of ill health that colonial Mexicans endured. So that we impose some kind of order over what is an otherwise haphazard collection of illnesses, we will start with the most clearly lethal diseases and work our way down to the less life-threatening ones. Our first foray into this world of sickness, then, will be the devastating epidemics that took so many lives, especially those of the native population in the first century of Spanish rule; next, we move on to the more common endemic illnesses that constituted an ever-present threat to the health of all *novohispanos*, or inhabitants of New Spain; and, finally, we end with a look at the everyday disorders that did not usually kill but proved to be, at best, troublesome nuisances and, at worse, extreme discomforts in this preanalgesic age.

"LA MAYOR LÁSTIMA DEL MUNDO"—EPIDEMIC ILLNESS

The terror and defenselessness that people of past centuries must have felt toward epidemic disease is difficult for most of us to imagine. At the beginning of the twenty-first century, those of us that live in the developed world probably think our chances of dying from an infectious disease are fairly remote. The battle against contagious diseases, which began to make real progress after the First World War, has had great success in identifying innumerable deadly microbes and controlling them through vaccination and the use of antibiotics. Because the majority of us no longer die from infectious diseases, we now live long enough to develop chronic illnesses such as cancer, heart-related ailments, and Alzheimer's disease, making these the most feared maladies of our time. Such trends are clearly seen in twentieth-century Mexico. In 1930, 47 percent of deaths resulted from infectious diseases, while only 10 percent of deaths were attributed to these causes in 1990; likewise, deaths due to problems in the circulatory system (primarily heart disease) rose from 1.9 percent to 19.8 percent in the same years.[17] The causes of these latest illnesses of civilization are closely linked to modern lifestyle—a surplus of cheap calories and increasingly inconvenient ways to burn them off—and the radically altered environment we live in; pathogens, although they may play a role in some cancers, are not viewed as significant factors in these diseases. In contrast, pathogens are still the most significant cause of morbidity and mortality in the developing world today. It is interesting to note that the one epidemic disease that has recently entered both the developed and developing worlds, AIDS, is viewed in the former as a disease of lifestyle—of homosexuals and drug users—even though most of its millions of victims in Africa and other parts of the developing world are neither. To view it as such is comforting because it implies that the individual has choices and thus control. Yet this sense of security, according to one researcher, may be a false one; the probability that new deadly diseases are awaiting the opportunity to invade the human species is great, with "AIDS appearing as merely the top of a viral iceberg."[18] The illusion of control also tends to obscure the importance that lethal microbes have played throughout human history, an experience well illustrated by the European conquest of the New World, where "far more Native Americans died in bed from Eurasian germs than on the battlefield from European guns and swords."[19]

The impact of Old World disease in the conquest of the New World is by now well known.[20] The initial contact with Europeans was catastrophic for native peoples of America, causing perhaps close to 90 percent loss of life in some areas within the first century after contact.[21] For the Valley of Mexico—the waterbound metropolis of Tenochtitlan-Tlateloco and other large settlements surrounding the lakes—estimates of depopulation in the sixteenth century range considerably. The largest estimate of population loss is as high as 97 percent, while the most conservative is about 60 percent.[22] Accurate figures probably fall somewhere in between these two extremes, but whatever the numbers, the scale of population loss, especially in the first half of the sixteenth century, was truly staggering. Epidemic disease was clearly the dominant factor in the rapid population decline, although the harsh treatment and ecological devastation that accompanied Spanish colonialization certainly magnified the losses.

New Spain suffered at least fifteen serious epidemics during the sixteenth century.[23] Three of these are mentioned frequently in contemporary Spanish and Nahuatl sources, indicating them to be the most serious and widespread of the century's pestilential outbreaks: the well-known smallpox epidemic of 1520–1, and the great epidemics of 1545–8 and 1576–80, either one, or both, of which could have been typhus. By all accounts, the most devastating was the smallpox epidemic of 1520–1, during the siege of Tenochtitlan, allegedly introduced by a black slave fighting with the Narváez contingent. The illness spread quickly within the city and outward to areas still unvisited by the Spaniards, killing hundreds of thousands. The enormous military significance played by the pestilence was evident to both native and European chroniclers of the conquest. Smallpox demolished the native elite, destroying their diplomatic and military capabilities just as Cortés was preparing his final onslaught on Tenochtitlan.[24]

The horror of this first pestilence comes through in several Nahua chronicles, the best-known of these being the account recorded by Sahagún in the *General History of the Things of New Spain*, his great encyclopedic enterprise on preconquest Nahua life. Book Twelve, a narration of the conquest, contains a vivid and melancholic description of the sufferers of smallpox:

> . . . at the time the Spaniards left Mexico, there came a great illness of pustules of which many local people died; it was called "the great rash" [totomanaliztli or huey zahuatl].
>
> . . . [The disease] brought great desolation: a great many died of it. They could no longer walk about, but lay in their dwellings and sleeping places, no longer able to move or stir. They were unable to change position, to stretch out on their sides or face down, or raise their heads. And when they made a motion, they called out loudly. The pustules that covered people caused great desolation; very many people died of them, and many just starved to death; starvation reigned, and no one took care of others any longer.
>
> On some people, the pustules appeared only far apart, and they did not suffer greatly, nor did many of them die of it. But many people's faces were spoiled by it, their faces were made rough. Some lost an eye or were blinded.[25]

The text is accompanied by drawings of people suffering with the disease. Reclining and wrapped in blankets, they are covered with pustules, their agony registered in their faces and body positions. One patient is crying out in pain, while another is receiving consolation from a woman. Unlike the Spanish accounts of indigenous experience with pestilence, which tend to be more impersonal and interpretive, this Nahua account—less filtered, more visceral—comes closer to capturing the horror of their experience. Besides the physical suffering and overwhelming death toll caused by the severity with which the illness struck, the psychological shock must have been overwhelming because nothing like that had ever happened to native Mexicans.

Smallpox is a horrific disease. It is extremely contagious; passed primarily through the air, a person can become infected just by inhaling a microscopic drop of the virus. Direct contact with any contaminated material, such as clothing or scabs, can also transmit the disease. After an incubation period of about twelve days, the victim develops a high fever, backache, vomiting, and severe malaise, followed shortly by the appearance of tiny red spots all over the body. These quickly turn into blisters, called pustules, which enlarge and eventually erupt as they become filled with pus. This eruption doesn't break the skin, but splits it horizontally, tearing away from its underlayers. The pain of the splitting is excruciating. At this point the patient either dies or the pustules dry up and form scabs which soon fall off, leaving disfiguring pox marks. It is believed that death is caused by a breathing arrest, a heart attack, shock, or a complete shutdown of the immune-system, but epidemiologist are still unsure how smallpox kills. The whole process takes about a month, after which a person is either dead or immune.[26] The two photographs of a British smallpox victim in 1896—one showing the man infected, the other showing him in health—gives those of us who have never seen or experienced this disease a more vivid impression of its brutal effects.

Mortality rates of this first epidemic can only be guessed at since contemporary estimates are crude and impressionistic. According to the friar Motolinía, one of the first Franciscans on the scene, "in some provinces half the people died, and in others a little less"; another Spaniard, a participant in the siege of Tenochtitlan, put the death rate at "more than one-fourth."[27] Because this was a "virgin-soil" epidemic, rates of infection could have been as high as 100 percent, with death rates of one-third or higher.[28] The severity of the smallpox epidemic of 1520–1 is easily explained by the New World's long isolation from the rest of mankind and evolutionary differences between the two areas in the development of pathogens. Pre-Columbian populations had no previous exposure to the crowd diseases that had forced the immunological systems of Old World peoples to erect defenses because they had completed their migration to the Americas by 10,000 BC, well before epidemic diseases had been established in the Old World. Throughout the course of conquest, the immunologically naïve inhabitants of the New World came in close contact with the "immunological supermen" of the Old World. Among the Europeans, it might be argued that the Iberians possessed one of the most evolved immunological systems in the world at that time. The peninsula had long been a crossroads of European and Arabic civilizations, and its roads had carried myriad peoples and their diseases for centuries. The cities of Iberia, where sewage and garbage flowed through the streets, abounded in disease-carrying rodents and insects; Iberians bathed infrequently, and their skin, hair, body fluids, and breath swarmed with pathogens. Exposed routinely to a host of childhood ailments, such as smallpox, measles, and mumps, their immunological systems indeed made them seem superhuman in the eyes of the natives being destroyed incomprehensibly by pestilence.[29]

The rise of epidemic disease in human history parallels the rise of civilizations. As long as humans lived in small isolated groups—nomadic hunter-gatherers, for example—their ailments were limited to chronic illnesses of low infectivity. Diseases that we tend to associate with large-scale epidemics, such as measles, smallpox, mumps, and pertussis can not sustain themselves in small populations. Lacking the essential antibodies, these groups could be wiped out entirely by an infected outsider, which in turn would kill the pathogens themselves, as they can only survive in the bodies of living people. Small population size helps explain not only why such groups could not sustain acute infectious diseases, but also why they could not evolve epidemic diseases of their own to give back to outsiders. In addition, small bands of hunter-gathers rarely remained in an area long enough to foul their water supplies and build up the refuse that would attract varmints that carry diseases and the vectors that spread them. Nor did these groups have the domesticated animals from which so many of the later crowd diseases originated. This is not to say that small human populations did not develop infectious disease. They did, but only of a certain type: those diseases in which the host can remain infected for a long time, such as amoebic dysentery, leprosy, and yaws, or those diseases that have microbes that can maintain themselves in alternative hosts, like water or insects, such as schistosomiasis or yellow fever. These groups were also susceptible to non-fatal infections to which humans do not develop lasting immunity like the common cold, flu, and internal parasites.[30]

Sedentary agriculture and the subsequent growth of cities expanded human populations to a density that could support very acute and very transient infections. Rapid transmission and acuteness are what give crowd diseases their terrible lethality. In a simplified form, epidemics work like this: microbes spread very rapidly within a local population, infecting almost everyone; victims either quickly die or recover and become immune, leaving no more infected people.

Because the microbes cannot survive except in human bodies, the disease dies out for the time being. With the birth of new and non-immune, generations, the local population again becomes susceptible to diseases carried by an infectious visitor from outside, thus starting a whole new epidemic cycle.[31]

The one-sidedness of the exchange of lethal pathogens between the Old and New Worlds is striking. Although over a dozen major infectious diseases were imported into the Americas by Europeans, perhaps not a single significant disease was passed to Europe from the New World. The one possible exception is syphilis, although its origins are still being debated. Yet, how is it possible that densely populated areas of the New World like Mesoamerica, the Andes, and the Mississippi Valley did not develop crowd diseases of their own? The most likely answer is that they had very few domesticated animals from which these diseases could evolve. Old World crowd diseases evolved out of the illnesses of herd animals that became domesticated; cattle, sheep, goats, dogs, pigs, horses, and fowl all contributed their pathogens to swelling pools of disease. People lived closely with these creatures, sharing water, air, and sometimes shelter with them. Thus, pox viruses were passed back and forth between humans and cattle to produce smallpox and cowpox, whereas the exchange and combination of different strains of viruses among dogs, cattle, and humans created distemper, rinderpest, and measles. The scarcity of domesticated animals in the Americas reflects the small number of wild animal candidates for domestication. Nearly 80 percent of its large wild mammals became extinct after the last Ice Age, about 13,000 years ago. Only five animals are known to have been domesticated in precontact America: the turkey in Mesoamerica, the guinea pig and llama/alpaca in the Andes, the Muscovy duck in tropical South America, and the dog throughout both continents. Yet none of these animals appear to have been likely sources of crowd diseases. Humans do not have much physical contact with Muscovy ducks and turkeys, nor do these fowl live in huge flocks. Guinea pigs, which do live closely among people, may have been the source of Chagas's disease or leishmaniasis, extremely unpleasant maladies, but not crowd killers. Nor did llamas and alpacas, the only comparable form of indigenous livestock found in the Americas, contribute to human disease pools, unlike cattle and sheep.[32] According to one researcher, the cameloids had four strikes against them as a source of human pathogens:

> [Llamas] were kept in smaller herds than were sheep and goats and pigs; their total numbers were never remotely as large as those of Eurasian populations of domestic livestock, since llamas never spread beyond the Andes; people don't drink (and get infected by) llama milk; and llamas aren't kept indoors, in close association with people. In contrast, human mothers in the New Guinea highlands often nurse piglets, and pigs as well as cows are frequently kept inside the huts of peasant farmers.[33]

Thus, the animal origins of human disease lie behind some of the broadest patterns of human history. For Native Americans, this chance aggregation of factors was momentous, as events in sixteenth-century Mexico so starkly demonstrate.

The smallpox epidemic of 1520–1 has become such a familiar component of the conquest narrative that subsequent epidemics tend to get slighted in the attention they get from historians. The two other major outbreaks of pestilence during the sixteenth century were probably as costly in terms of human life as the first one and had equally dire consequences for the indigenous communities that suffered them. Spanish writers who witnessed the epidemics of 1545–8 and 1576–80 were astounded by the tremendous number of dead.[34] Sahagún writes:

> In the year 1545 there was a huge and universal pestilence where, in all of New Spain, most of the people who lived there died. At the time of this pestilence I was in Mexico City, in the part of Tlateloco, and I buried more than 10,000 bodies, and at the end of the pestilence I became ill and almost died.[35]

Indigenous sources chronicle these events as a great *cocoliztle,* (great plague or illness) in various codices. The *Códice Telleriano-Remensis,* for example, records the epidemic of 1545–8 with paintings of cadavers wrapped in straw mats and bundled together. Linked by lines to glifs representing those years, the accompanying gloss states: "[in the] year of 1544 and of 1545 there was a great mortality among the Indians."[36]

The epidemic of 1576–80 is especially rich in documentation; for a variety of reasons, many reports were compiled around this time, so mention of it is common. Several of the *Relaciones Geográficas* offer commentary about the epidemic and its destructive effects on a population already reeling from more than fifty years of contact with European diseases. The *Relación de Cuauhiquilpan,* for example, states that ". . . in this pueblo there are very few Indians at the present time: there used to be more than five hundred Indians of tribute, but about four years ago many died of the pestilence, so that now it seems no more than fifty remain."[37] A sudden drop in population had far-reaching consequences in the new colony; it meant that there were no longer people available to work the fields and orchards, and many communities fell into ruin. Antonio de Ciudad Real, traveling during the years 1584–9 through Mexico with Fray Alonso Ponce, a Franciscan commissary-general, notes how one community was reduced to ruin by the epidemic:

> In times past that town had a large population, according to the older people and now it just seems like ruins of houses, and for the many fruit trees there are in the

surroundings, among which the Indians usually have their towns, especially being in the hot lands, like it is, but with the *cocolitzle,* there was such a very large pestilence and mortality in that land, that everything was destroyed and now there are scarcely two hundred inhabitants.[38]

The impression that things had fallen into a state of disintegration was widespread throughout all of New Spain. Spaniards, for the most part, were spared from these early epidemics, but they must have been truly shaken as they watched their labor force die off like flies ("como chinches" said one source).[39] One of the most poignant descriptions of this experience comes from a letter written during the epidemic by a hacienda owner to an acquaintance in Spain. His estate has fallen into a state of idleness for lack of workers, and he appears frightened and overwhelmed by the magnitude of death he sees around him. The pestilence, he says, is "*la mayor lástima del mundo,*" the greatest sorrow of the world.

> . . . at the present time there has been and still is a pestilence among the natives so widespread and so terrible that it is the greatest sorrow of the world, and in the province of Tlaxcala, where I live, they say that more than 80,000 people have died, and at our hacienda we have lost more than 200 people, and among those some blacks, and for this the work of the hacienda has stopped and we are all trying to do what we can, giving orders to find people, but none can be found. . . . God in his mercy has guarded the Spaniards, because until now only a few of them have died, but we are in great fear . . . and so everyone here is with great necessity, because the wealth of this land are these Indians, because, as there are so many, they provide service and work, and as so many of them have died, everything has stopped.[40]

What diseases could have caused such staggering population loss? Various modern scholars, beginning with Alexander Von Humboldt at the turn of the nineteenth century, have sought the answer to this question, but no clear consensus has emerged. The identification of diseases from historical descriptions is a dubious task. Specialists usually have to work from contemporary records of symptoms, which can be a problem since descriptions are often vague and in many cases the same symptom could result from different illnesses. Even for the most clearly and widely described illnesses, such as smallpox or typhus, it is often difficult to make an exact diagnosis because the circumstances that favor the spread of one type of illness can create opportunities for the transmission of another, thus creating multiple epidemics in a community at the same time. This, in turn, frequently produces a confusing record of symptoms.[41] Humboldt identified the pestilence in 1545–8 as *matlazáhuatl,* a Nahua term that came to be associated with typhus sometime after the middle of the sixteenth century.[42]

Other scholars appear more skeptical about assigning an identity to this epidemic. Contemporary sources, both Spanish and indigenous, failed to call the disease by any name, neither *tabardillo*—the Spanish name for typhus—nor *matlazáhuatl*.[43] Mendieta, for example, wrote that both epidemics were due to "*pujamiento de sangre*," or "full bloodiness," but that the illness of 1576 was also *tabardillo*.[44] One of the most striking symptoms recorded for both epidemics was bleeding from the nose. The *Códice de 1576*, for example, states: "In August came the pestilence, blood came from our noses, we made our confessions to the friars and they gave us permission to eat meat, the doctors cured us." One of the illustrations accompanying the Nahuatl text shows a person bleeding copiously from the nose.[45]

Other symptoms are vividly described in the *Relación de Ocopetlayuca*, a small *corregimiento* located on the southern slope of Popocatépetl in the present-day state of Puebla, which lost over a third of its inhabitants in the 1576–80 epidemic. An eyewitness reports that:

> . . . it is the nature of this illness that it causes great pain in the "mouth of the stomach" with horrible fever in all parts of the body and head, and those that die, do so within six or seven days; . . . the ones that survive become healthy, although sometimes the illness attacks them again and they die. No medicine is effective against this disease.[46]

That this was an outbreak of typhus is further suggested by later comparisons of it to another severe epidemic, that of the great *matlazáhuatl* epidemic of 1736.[47] But an accurate diagnosis of the illnesses behind these epidemics may never be known. Sources fail to mention the rash that is characteristic of typhus, and the most conspicuous symptom reported, bleeding from the nose, does not figure among presently known symptoms of the disease. Yet the magnitude of death in both epidemics has made typhus a plausible explanation because its potential lethality is as great as smallpox, measles, or plague, any of which would have been easily recognized at this time.

Like smallpox, typhus can be an extremely acute illness in its epidemic form. In a typical course, onset can begin abruptly with a very high fever, severe headache, extreme weakness, and general malaise. A rash appears on the fourth or fifth day, usually starting on the shoulders and trunk, and sometimes spreading to the extremities, although it rarely appears on the face. This is not a blistery rash, like that of smallpox, but one of barely raised spots, ranging from two to five millimeters in diameter. Both its Nahuatl and Spanish names refer to its distinguishing rash: *matlazáhuatl*, a composite of *matatl*, meaning "net," and *záhuatl*, indicating "eruptions" or "rash," thus a "net-like rash"; and *tabardillo* (or sometimes *tabardete*) in reference to the rash covering the body like a "tabard," or sleeveless cloak. In fatal episodes, the patient becomes completely debilitated, falls into a coma, and dies of cardiac arrest; mortality rates can be as high as 25 percent. In contrast to the smallpox virus, which cannot survive outside living human bodies, typhus is transmitted to people by insects. Several of the Old World epidemic diseases transferred to the Americas were spread by anthropoids such as lice, fleas, and mosquitoes. Malaria and yellow fever—both well-known illnesses spread by mosquitoes—have been endemic, and sometimes epidemic, in many parts of tropical America since the sixteenth century. The port of Vera Cruz, for example, was a dreaded stop for travelers because of its seasonal outbreaks of yellow fever. Like the bubonic form of plague, the typhus virus is carried by rats in their fleas, which explains how the disease persists between outbreaks. Humans can contract the endemic form of typhus from the bites of rat fleas. An epidemic results when people begin to transmit the virus among themselves, which happens if they are infested with body lice. The body and the head louse, which travel easily among people in crowded conditions, take up the virus from the infected blood of one victim, and leave it on the skin of another by way of their feces. The virus enters the body through abrasions in the skin, such as scratched insect bites, and the process of infection begins its cycle. Typhus confers an immunity on its survivors, which, though not permanent, may last for years. Early modern Spaniards only became familiar with the epidemic form of typhus at the end of the fifteenth century, when it first appeared during the battle for Granada in 1489–90. Hans Zinsser, who wrote a history of typhus during the 1930s, believed that the disease was brought to Spain by soldiers from Cyprus, where it was prevalent. It struck the Iberian Peninsula repeatedly during the sixteenth century, and it gradually spread to the rest of Europe, assisted chiefly by the march of armies. Just how and when typhus entered the New World is still not known, but in all likelihood it was transported by infected rats aboard ships from Spain.[48]

Epidemic diseases periodically assaulted the inhabitants of Mexico throughout the colonial period and well into the nineteenth century, although the extent of population loss during subsequent epidemics was never as great as in the sixteenth-century episodes. The one exception may be the great epidemic of *matlazáhuatl* of 1736–9, where it was estimated by an eyewitness that more than a third of the inhabitants of Mexico died.[49] In addition to smallpox and typhus, measles, mumps, scarlet fever, whopping cough, and yellow fever all remained endemic in parts of New Spain between their periodic appearances as pestilence. These highly contagious diseases, very often referred to simply as "*la peste*," were the most feared by all sections of the population, regardless of their social class or race. The ex-voto of Doña Luisana, with which I opened this chapter, not only gives us a pictographic starting point for imaging the experience of a smallpox victim, but also poignantly affirms the old adage that every statistic conceals real personal misfortune. During the years 1761–2, most of New Spain had been in the grip of smallpox and typhus, which had swept through the colony killing thousands. No firm mortality rates are known but one contemporary estimate put the death toll in Mexico City alone at around 25,000 people.[50] The date of Doña Luisana's ex-voto, the winter of 1761, confirms she was part of this epidemic, and her location, Cholula, a city just outside of Puebla, would have placed her in a densely populated area of Mexico, where infectious diseases could freely run their course. The painted scene portrays the sufferer as an upper class woman; although the room is simple, the sick-bed appears to be outfitted with costly, decorative linens and the people attending the patient are dressed quite formally, especially the men. Doña Luisana "being sick from smallpox, and very dangerously so," languishes in her sick-bed, her skin completely covered with a frightful rash, although she appears to be well attended by caregivers. That this sufferer survived her ordeal is evident from the ex-voto itself, as it was produced to show gratitude for "the marvels" the divine images in it bestowed on the patient.[51] This ex-voto is vivid testimony that *la peste* was a category of illness to be feared above all else, a sentiment also poignantly expressed in letters the Condesa de Miravalle wrote to her son-in-law, Pedro Romero de Terreros, around this time. She implores her family to be mindful of their diet and extra vigilant about guarding the children's health, . . . "the epidemic raging here, which spreads wherever it enters and leaves no one alive, is worse than the smallpox."[52]

There is little doubt that epidemic disease (with the possible exception of infant mortality) was responsible for most premature deaths throughout the history of New Spain. Frequently these were "compound epidemics" in which the appearance of one disease triggered others latent in the population, creating a combination of disease agents with often disastrous results. These pestilential invasions, for which there were no known effective treatments, were so varied in character, and so widely dispersed in time and space that all inhabitants, white or native, rich or poor, young or old, were threatened by them at some time in their lives. The bulk of epidemic victims, however, were disproportionately from the lower groups in the socioeconomic order—in New Spain, this meant the vast majority of the population, almost all of them Indians and mestizos. This ancient affinity between poverty and disease was intensified by the fact that epidemics frequently ran in cycles that paralleled widespread crop failures, generating the twin scourges of sickness and famine.[53] Over the years, various lists have been compiled of these pestilential crises. Writing in the eighteenth century, Cayetano Cabrera y Quintero chronicles eighteen major epidemics from 1520 to 1737, and notes the extremely high mortality rate among Indians, for which he attributes their poverty, excessive drinking of *pulque*, and an intense fatalism in the face of death. Gibson's list of colonial epidemics is extensive: apart from fifteen in the sixteenth century, he catalogs thirty-five more for the remainder of the colonial period.[54]

In the last century of colonial rule, smallpox erupted into epidemic form every fifteen to twenty years, with enormous loss of life. In 1798, the Spanish king, Charles IV, ordered a massive vaccination campaign for all of Spain's colonies, and, in 1804, Jenner's vaccine became available in Mexico for the first time. Popular acceptance of the new procedure was widespread and mortality was greatly reduced, but in the turbulent nineteenth century, vaccination campaigns were practiced intermittently, thus ensuring that smallpox would not be eradicated from Mexican soil for another century and a half.[55] Unfortunately, at the turn of the nineteenth century, the same optimistic prospects did not hold true for that other killer of the colonial period, the louse-borne disease of typhus. This is not surprising given the inadequacies of public and private hygiene practices of the time and the state of medical knowledge, which still did not fully understand the causal relationship between filth and disease.

"QUEBRANTADA DE SALUD":—ENDEMIC ILLNESS

Although epidemics show up as distinct peaks of mortality in the historical record, making them fairly visible to the researcher, the range and scale of endemic disease is more difficult to discern. Yet colonial sources are full of testimonies about the more frequent illnesses afflicting people, especially those that manifested themselves with gastrointestinal symptoms. One chronicler noted that as Fray Alonso Ponce was making his way, on foot and horseback, through New Spain during the 1580s, he was overcome by "vomiting, so severe and of such quantity of black humor, that the official [he was traveling with] became terrified." When asked to record which diseases were most prevalent in the towns of New Spain, the authors of the *Relaciones Geográficas* cited *cámeras de sangre* ("bloody diarrhea") more than any other illness. And, in a letter she wrote in July 1757, the Condesa de Miravalle remarked to her son-in-law that she was "*bien quebantada*," that is, her health was "broken" as she had just endured an episode of "dark vomit" and now was suffering from a severe cough.[56] Colonial Mexicans mention *los vómitos* and *las cámeras* so often in their writings, there can be little doubt that gastrointestinal ailments were the most ubiquitous of maladies. Equally universal, too, were the illnesses that involved the respiratory system; then, as now, everyone suffered their fair share of head colds, coughs, *mal de pecho*, and sore throats, along with more serious respiratory ailments. Although these two sets of symptoms, gastrointestinal and respiratory, could stem from any number of diseases, many of them deadly, they often were viewed as illnesses in and of themselves.

Juan de Cárdenas, writing in the sixteenth century on various aspects of the people and animals born in the Indies, comments on the ubiquity of stomach problems in New Spain. "Certainly . . . in the Indies, there is scarcely a man that does not go around complaining of his stomach, no matter whether he be old or young, man or woman, born in the Indies, or recently arrived from Spain . . ."[57] This same observation is made by Fray Agustín Farfán, a doctor who wrote a popular book on domestic medicine late in the sixteenth century. His first chapter is devoted to *flaqueza de estomago* ("weakness of the stomach"). Like Cárdenas, Farfán notes the many people who seem to suffer from this malady: "It is very sad to see in New Spain the many that complain of weak stomach, and of not being able to digest their food, even when they have eaten little."[58] Both authors were writing about the Spanish population of New Spain which seems to have suffered from an array of gastrointestinal problems. Farfán is very specific in his descriptions of the symptoms:

> Some eat what appeals to them and what their stomachs desires, even though they can not digest it. Others vomit what they eat along with a great quantity of putrid and acidic humors. Others throw up and belch gas all day long, and spit up phlegm and they vomit curds that are clear like egg whites.[59]

Just why Europeans would have endured a myriad of digestive problems is given a great deal of attention in both these works, and rightly so as the stomach played a pivotal role in the humoral view of how the body worked, something that will be explored in chapter four of this book. New immigrants would have undoubtedly encountered a host of gastroenteric pathogens to which they would have had no immunity, causing them stomach problems and diarrhea just as modern travelers do today. Many Spanish emigrants in their letters to family and friends back in Spain complain of being sick. Alonso de Alocer, writing to his brother in Madrid complains: ". . . since coming here I have not had one day of health, because everyone that comes here from Spain gets *chapetonada* and more than a third of those that come die of it." The *chapetón* (recently arrived Spaniard), was vulnerable to sudden illness and death, as many of these letters confirm. One letter writer informs an acquaintance in Jaén that his brother in Mexico City has died suddenly from diarrhea, whereas another informs her daughter in Sevilla that "God has been served" by taking the life of her husband, who died from "diarrhea, along with fever."[60]

Diseases of the respiratory tract also were prevalent. Contemporaries called these illnesses by a variety of names: *romadizo, catarro, tos, tos antiqua, pasmo, hinchazones en la garganta*, and *asma*. More serious respiratory infections were also common. One that is mentioned in many of the domestic medicine manuals and in contemporary descriptions of illness is *dolor de costado*, literally, "pain in the side." Both Farfán and Esteyneffer describe this disease by listing its most common symptoms: the patient feels a very sharp pain in one of his sides, has a high fever, has great difficulty breathing, a persistent cough, and "hard" pulse. "When all these symptoms and signals are present," writes Farfán, "then *dolor de costado* is very dangerous, and can kill quickly, depending on the state of the patient." He later states that the first thing an attending physician should do is to make sure the patient has made confession and has "put his soul in order."[61] Juan de Brihuega, an inhabitant of Puebla in the sixteenth century, almost lost his pregnant wife to this disease; she was so sick that "they bled her six times, and because of this, she almost died."[62] *Dolor de costado* must have specified a large group of symptoms common to many actual diseases, such as pleurisy, emphysema, pneumonia, or tuberculosis.

People often simply described their illnesses by it most prominent symptom, *calentura*, or fever. In the town of Cuicatlán, the Indians tend mostly to be sick from "fevers, because it is very hot there . . ." and in the nearby pueblo of Tututepetongo, "they sometimes get some fevers, which they cure with wild maguey leaves."[63] Both the Nahua and European medical systems recognized different types and qualities of fevers; contemporaries called them by various names: *tercianas, cuartanas, calentura hética, calentura continua*. Marco Ortiz wrote to his father in 1569 that he had been very ill "with chills and double tertian fever (*tercianas dobles*) that lasted for six months, [after which] I was cured, God being served." Antonio de Ciudad Real happily notes the day, in *Tratado curioso*, when he realized that he was finally free from quartan fever (*cuartanas*), which had plagued him for more than three years.[64] Intermittent fevers like these were probably malarial, and these two cases could very well have originated in Spain, as their carriers had only recently arrived from the Peninsula. Each of the different species of malarial parasites have their own periodicity. For example, the parasite causing benign tertian malaria, *Plasmodium viva*, has an incubation time of about ten to seventeen days; the resulting fever, which can be as high as 104–106 degrees Fahrenheit, lasts for two to six hours and recurs every third day. In contrast, the incubation period for quartan malaria, caused by *Plasmodium malariae*, can be as long as thirty or forty days, with fever coming every fourth day. These episodes of fever are usually accompanied by nausea, vomiting, diarrhea, and, at the end of the attack, profuse sweating. Both types of malaria, if left untreated, can last for months; as the disease progresses, the spleen enlarges, and the patient becomes anemic and sometimes jaundiced.[65] That malaria was present in New Spain is well known—it proved quite destructive to coastal Indians in the early colonial period—but whether it preceded the Spaniards is still a matter of dispute. Those well-versed in precontact medicine say that the Nahuas were familiar with intermittent fevers and came to distinguish them by their pattern of onset and recurrence.[66]

Another mosquito-borne illness that claimed many victims in the colonial and early national period was yellow fever. Endemic in the coastal areas of Mexico until its eradication in the early 1920s, this disease, which could well have been the "Montezuma's Revenge" of its day for the way it seemed to attack only Europeans, is forever linked to the history of Veracruz. As the region's only serviceable port, the coastal city was established soon after the conquest, not as a desirable location of Spanish settlement, but as a necessary link between New Spain and the outside world. Shortly thereafter, inbound Spanish passengers, who had no choice but to pass through the insalubrious city, were calling this place *la tumba de los españoles*, for its horrible association with pestilential fevers. By the eighteenth century, travelers and residents alike attributed the many deaths to one disease in particular: *el vómito prieto*, or as it came to be known in the late colonial period, *fiebre amarilla*.[67] One traveler, the indefatigable Capuchine friar, Francisco de Ajofrín, had this to say about the horrors of the illness:

> The terrible disease that has been suffered by this city (although now somewhat alleviated) is the "black vomit," which is vomit of black blood and putrefaction. This formidable contagious disease, which has buried in an infinite number of Europeans, does not bother the Indians with any regularity, and so it really belongs to those who come from the other side. . . . The first signs of this illness is the vomit itself and symptoms so mortal and expeditious, that many die on the first day; others, on the second or third; it being rare that any escape; nor have the study and effort of many doctors and surgeons, of the fleets or shore, [who have] examined this disease with great diligence, been able to find any medicine to prevent or cure it.[68]

Although the symptoms of yellow fever can be quite mild—some victims recover unaware of ever having contracted the disease—the more serious forms can be horrific and life-threatening. Nausea, high fever, and severe headache set in usually three to six days after the initial infection. As the disease advances, the liver becomes damaged, causing the two most distinctive indications of yellow fever: jaundice and bleeding from the gums, nasal passages, and stomach lining, which is exacerbated by the liver's inability to make essential factors needed by the body's blood-clotting system. The severe gastrointestinal bleeding causes frequent, and at times violent, hematemesis (vomiting of blood), and it was this symptom that earned the sickness the name of *vómito prieto*. Among these more serious cases, mortality can be as high as 50 percent. Death comes quickly after the appearance of renal failure, convulsions, and cardiovascular collapse, usually seven to ten days after the initial onset of symptoms.[69]

If the phenomenon of Indians succumbing to smallpox while Spaniards were unaccountably spared was baffling to contemporaries, equally mystifying was the way in which yellow fever struck Europeans while the native population remained largely unaffected. In the nineteenth century, Southerners in the United States referred to this same illness as the "stranger's disease" because it appeared to attack only visitors from the northern states or Europe while inexplicably sparing long-term residents, both blacks and whites. In Veracruz, lifelong residents had little to fear from yellow fever, which seemed solely to afflict recent arrivals on the incoming ships or highlanders descending to the coastal region. This occurred because the city provided a perfect conflux of disease-prone conditions. The heavy rainfall and year-round warm temperatures offered an ideal environment for a thriving mosquito population; the two types known to carry the yellow fever virus in Latin America, *Haemagogus* and *Aedes aegypti*, flourished here.[70] According to one historian, Veracruz itself provided a perfect setting for the latter, which breeds preferentially in small bodies and containers of water.

> Drainage in the rain-soaked town was notoriously poor. Heavy showers left alleyways and plazas inundated with water for days, even weeks. Street puddles combined with household pots and vases and the large cisterns that stored drinking water in wealthier homes to give the periodomestic mosquito ample opportunity to spawn during the wet summer months.[71]

Longtime residents of areas where yellow fever is endemic are unlikely to experience dramatic outbreaks of the disease because exposure early in life, usually resulting in milder cases of infection, confers immunity from later infection. Yet, as New Spain's only Atlantic port, Veracruz's streets were frequently filled with a large susceptible host population. Each year, the Spanish *flota* brought hundreds of immigrants with no prior exposure to the yellow fever virus, along with scores of equally vulnerable highland residents who descended to meet them and the goods brought by the ships. And, after 1778, when Charles III liberalized colonial trade laws, the economic opportunities in Veracruz attracted newcomers from both sides of the Atlantic. Thousands of *comerciantes*, peddlers, artisans, day laborers, muleteers, and sailors from Spain and the interior of Mexico entered the mosquito-infested harbor with little or no immunity from the virus. That *vómito prieto* would infect hundreds, if not thousands, of people almost every year was virtually assured by one more factor in this convergence of conditions: seasonal weather patterns in the gulf coast. Because of their breeding and lifespan cycles, the mosquito population reached its peak in August and September, well after the onset of summer rains. Coinciding with this infestation were the arrivals of the ships from Spain. The *flota* bound for

Mexico left Seville in early to mid-summer, crossed the Atlantic via the Canaries, and entered the port of Veracruz in late summer or early fall, usually just in time to avoid hurricane season and the arrival of the northern winds, *los nortes*, that made navigation in the gulf so treacherous.[72]

The cycle of sickness that descended on Veracruz every year ended rather abruptly in late fall as the northern winds literally swept the threat of disease from the port. Because *aedes aegypti* is a weak flier, strong winds can push the mosquitoes far from their preferred habitat.[73] The arrival of the *nortes* coincided with the end of the rainy season, curtailing the breeding of any remaining mosquitoes until a new cycle could begin the following spring.

Although the more visible infectious diseases produced high levels of morbidity and mortality in the colonial population, other illnesses, of great consequences but less visible as causes of death, also took their toll. Modern paleopathological analysis of skeletons disinterred from beneath the Metropolitan Cathedral of Mexico City have revealed some interesting data on the health of colonial inhabitants. In addition to the more predictable findings, such as the prevalence of osteoarthritis, osteomyelitis, and many bone fractures caused by trauma, the study revealed a surprisingly high incidence of two diseases: scurvy and syphilis.[74]

Scurvy, a disease caused by a lack of vitamin C, was first recognized to be a major problem for Europeans in the late fifteenth century, a period that coincided with technological advances in shipbuilding that allowed for very long sea voyages. Because the human body cannot produce ascorbic acid endogenously, it is completely dependent on dietary sources—mainly fresh fruit and vegetables, and to a much lesser extent, fresh meat—for the vitamin. Salted or dried meats (these curing methods result in the loss of the vitamin), grains, nuts, eggs, and dairy products provide little or no vitamin C. Scurvy is a serious disease, one that can easily kill its victim if left untreated. The lack of ascorbic acid impairs the body's ability to manufacture collagen, an essential glycoprotein component of connective tissue. Scurvy first appears in vitamin-deficient individuals in about twelve weeks, causing extreme fatigue and lethargy. After some seventeen to twenty-six weeks without consumption of vitamin C, the more severe symptoms set in: hemorrhagic spots under the skin, softening of the gums, and defective wound healing. The traditional diet on long voyages—wheat flour, salted meat, oatmeal, dried peas, oil, and cheese—was almost totally lacking in vitamin C. By the end of the fifteenth century, long-distance travel by sea had become more common, meaning that people could now stay at sea for months at a time, long enough to suffer the deleterious effects of not having an adequate supply of fresh fruits and vegetables. One researcher has estimated that at least one million seamen died from this disease between the years 1600, when long voyages had become more common, and 1800, when the protective effects of lemon juice became known. "In this sense scurvy . . . may truly be regarded as one of the earliest occupational diseases."[75]

The effects of scurvy, or *escorbuto*, on seamen are vividly described by Antonio de la Ascension, a priest who accompanied an expedition from Mexico in 1602 to explore the coastline of California. When the ship was delayed by adverse winds, the crew members began to develop some alarming symptoms, such as body aches, large purple spots covering the body, severe stiffening of the legs and thighs, extreme swelling of the gums "to such a size that neither the teeth nor the molars can be brought together . . . [and] the teeth become so loose and without support that they move while moving the head." With this disease, the victims "come to be so weakened . . . that their natural vigor fails them, and they die all of a sudden, while talking." The writer also noted that the mysterious disease broke out in the same place that the Spanish fleet, coming back from the Philippines to Mexico each year, experienced the same problem. He concluded that the winds of that area are "so sharp, subtle and cold" that they "pass through thin men." These winds, he continued, carry with them "much pestilence, and if in itself the air is not bad, it produces with its subtlety and coldness some corruption of bad humors, especially in persons worn out and fatigued with the hardships of the navigation." Some of the crew survived the trip to California because a forced landing was made in Mazatlan where some of the ship's members discovered a cactus fruit that grew in abundance there. The acidic fruit, along with the efforts of the Virgin del Monte Carmel, restored the health of those on board fairly quickly.[76]

Although evidence of scurvy was most clearly seen among sailors on long voyages, it should be remembered that it also affected early modern urban populations; the inhabitants of European cities frequently suffered from this malady.[77] That evidence of scurvy was found in skeletal remains from the Cathedral's cemetery is understandable when we recall that only people of Spanish origin are likely to have been buried there. Most *criollos*—the American-born descendants of Spanish immigrants—were urban residents and probably had diets that lacked a variety of fresh fruits and vegetables a good deal of the time. During the colonial years, too, *escorbuto* was often associated with dental conditions and with venereal disease. One remedy from the eighteenth century, advertised in the *Gaceta de Mexico*, promised to "clean, whiten, and fortify the teeth," and also to cure scurvy. Another praised the virtues of two types of agave plants that were useful in the treatment of venereal disease and scurvy, and "other diseases which do not respond to the use of mercury and other known remedies."[78]

There is much evidence that syphilis was also a major health problem among New Spain's population, especially in the sixteenth century when, because of its newness, the disease struck with a virulence it was to lose in later centuries. If sufferers of *bubas*, as the disease was then commonly called, were thick on the ground in the new colony, so were a myriad of healers peddling remedies for this affliction. In 1527, one of the first acts of the new *Ayuntamiento* was to issue an order prohibiting unlicensed practitioners from treating "those that are sick with *bubas* and other sores or pains . . . on penalty of sixty gold pesos for each time done to the contrary."[79] In the 1540s, the bishop Juan de Zumárraga erected the *Hospital del Amor de Dios* primarily to care for syphilitics; the medical staff of eighteen included four *untadores*—people who applied the mercurial unguents that were the standard treatment of the day.[80] Medical writers in the sixteenth century seemed particularly interested in this disease—its origins, its bewildering variety of symptoms, and its treatments, especially those coming out of the New World. Pedro Arias de Benavides devoted almost his entire *Secretos de cirugía* to the diagnosis and treatment of *morbo gálico*, the French disease, which was the other favored appellation of the time. In his treatise on medicine, Farfán expressed "great sorrow for those I see each day who die of the sickness of *bubas*"; he warns his readers there are many who claim to know how to cure this illness, but end up leaving their patients "worse than when they began the cure." He continues with advice on how to recognize and treat the disease with various substances and techniques such as sarsaparilla, guaiacum, various ointments, and fumigation. Juan de Cárdenas, in his typically florid language, also had much to say about the disease; his claim that syphilis was more widespread in New Spain than anywhere else in the world is certainly hyperbolic, but does give a sense of the magnitude of the problem.

> Among the diseases, because of our recent faults and recent sins, that have lately found and tested the human body, one of them, the Indies disease, or, according to others, the French disease, is so infernally malignant and pernicious, that it truly afflicts, oppresses, and torments men, without any exception. It is now even commonly said in the Indies that one is not an honored man if he does not carry in his face a sign or trace of this sickness. Thus, it is so bleak [to see] the use of the black velvet patch for the face, a bump on the temple, a sign of bone lacking in the forehead, that one no longer dares to look; so that if we were to meticulously ponder, and notice the broken color [of the face], the little pains in the joints, the small blisters and sores around the mouth . . . we could go on forever; but at last we are able to cleanly extract our proposition, which is the certain and well examined conclusion, that there is no other province or kingdom in the world where this disease afflicts more, nor where more mercury, guaiacum, *china*, and sarsaparilla are consumed . . . [81]

The reference to bumps, blisters, and pains in the joints are just some of the more common symptoms that were recorded by chroniclers in the sixteenth century. The surgeon Arias describes the signs of *morbo gálico* as sores on the penis, swellings in the groin area, pains in the joints, the loss of hair, especially the eyebrows and eyelashes, sores in the mouth, bad digestion, headaches without fever, bumps on the head, very bad color in the face, and "weakness, such that they are too tired to walk and desire to sit and do not want to get up again."[82] Bernal Díaz tells us that many of Cortés's soldiers had trouble descending the steep stairs of the Aztec temple in Tenochtitlan because "they were suffering from *bubas* or humors, and it hurt their muscles to walk down."[83] The name *bubas* comes from the distinctive sores and swellings that appear on all parts of the body, including the skin of the palms and soles, and in the mouth as well as around the genitalia and the anus. Today, we know that these symptoms are characteristic of secondary syphilis, which sets in about six weeks after the primary sore, or chancre, appears on the genitals. After the secondary symptoms heal and disappear, there is a latent period, which can last many years, during which time the treponemes that cause the disease lurk in the tissues and intermittently in the blood and spinal fluid. During this time, the sufferer may be free of symptoms. Late, or tertiary, syphilis displays itself with the onset of more serious, even life-threatening, complications: the destruction of bone; inflammation of the heart and blood vessels, the eyes, or central nervous system; and lastly, syphilis can attack the brain itself, creating extreme dementia, even insanity.[84] That this dreadful disease revealed itself in three different stages was not known until the middle of the nineteenth century when the French venereologist, Philippe Ricord, described the natural progression of the illness.[85]

The variety of symptoms described by observers and sufferers in its early days underscores the need to be cautious about drawing too rigid a picture of the disease, which clearly changed over the years. In its first decades of existence, there is evidence that the malady was quite malignant and deadly. Like any infectious disease that is introduced into a population with little or no immunity, the classic course of the illness is rapid spread and extreme virulence, followed later by diminishing severity. Descriptions of the malady from the late fifteenth and early sixteenth centuries relate the horror of its effects: the terrible sores and swellings, often extending into the mouth and throat, and leaving the body covered with scabs that turned from red to black; severe fever; pain in the bones so intense that patients "screamed day and night without respite, envying the dead themselves"; and, often early death. By the seventeenth century, however, syphilis had likely become the disease we know it to be today: a very dangerous infection, but not one that would "be called explosive in the nature of its attack on the victim."[86] It is also important to remember that *bubas* was sometimes used as a catch-all term to denote a wide collection of symptoms. Syphilis, in some of its dermatologic manifestations, resembles leprosy; and, as Esteyneffer notes, *bubas* and scurvy are sometimes confused because their pains in the joints and bones are similar. Furthermore, individuals could be infected with more than one disease, or more than one venereal disease, at a time, accounting for a sometimes bewildering mixture of physical symptoms. Given these circumstances, it would be difficult for even a sophisticated diagnostician to make an accurate inference about the identity and natural course of the illness.[87]

The historiography of syphilis is vast and its origins have been debated since its first appearance in Western Europe in the last decade of the fifteenth century. Alfred Crosby has noted the special fascination this illness holds for historians, which he attributes to its abrupt beginnings:

> . . . of all mankind's most important maladies, it is the most uniquely "historical." The beginnings of most diseases lie beyond man's earliest rememberings. Syphilis, on the other hand, has a beginning. Many men, since the last decade of the fifteenth century, have insisted that they knew almost exactly when syphilis appeared on the world stage and even where it came from.[88]

Among the early chroniclers of the disease, there is a broad consensus that it first appeared in Italy sometime between the years 1494–6 when King Charles VII of France led an attack against the Kingdom of Naples. His army was made up of about 30,000 men—mostly mercenaries, including some from Spain—and, like most armies of the day, was accompanied by an assortment of civilians, including hundreds of prostitutes. When the invaders were finally ejected by King Alphonso II with the help of Spanish mercenaries sent by Ferdinand and Isabella, they continued to spread the disease far and wide as they returned to their own countries. Charles himself died of syphilis in 1498. By this time, with the disease raging throughout continental Europe, it was estimated that about 20 percent of the population was infected with what was now being called the French disease.[89]

Controversy about whether syphilis existed in the Old World before the return of Columbus from the New World has continued from the early sixteenth century to our own time. The vast accumulation of documentary materials and, since the late nineteenth century, new evidence from the evolving field of paleopathology has had the effect of extending, rather than settling, the debate. Although proponents of an American origin for the disease cite some persuasive evidence to back up their theory, a large part of their argument rests on the conspicuous *lack* of evidence that syphilis ever existed anywhere on the Eurasian continent: first, no unequivocal description of it has ever been found in written sources predating the late fifteenth century, none, that is, that would clearly distinguish it from diseases with similar symptoms such as leprosy or scabies, a fact hard to ignore for a disease that spreads as widely and as quickly as syphilis does wherever people are exposed to it; and, second, no human remains dating from before the 1490s showing signs of syphilitic damage have ever been found in the countless excavations of Old World civilizations. This striking absence of any sign of Old World origins is bolstered by some documentary evidence from the early years of the Spanish empire and a steadily growing collection of physical evidence indicating American provenance. Nearly a generation after the Colombian voyages, medical men and historians began insisting that the new disease was brought back to Europe by Columbus's crew in 1493. Both Bartolomé de las Casas and Gonzalo Fernández de Oviedo y Valdés, two of the most important early chroniclers of Spanish America, and each with personal experience and access to people who sailed with Columbus, argued that the disease was clearly imported into Europe by the first voyagers to return from the New World. Their claim was backed up by others, including Columbus's son, Ferdinand, and a Spanish physician named Ruy Díaz de Isla who claimed that he had treated some of the sailors for an unknown disease whose symptoms later turned out to be those of *morbo gálico.* Even more persuasive then such claims are the growing number of physical remains excavated from American soil. Precontact skeletons showing syphilitic damage have been identified by paleopathologists, bolstering the argument that treponemal diseases, including syphilis, existed in New World populations. Another theory complicating this debate is one that holds that treponemal diseases had long been present in the Old World prior to the epidemic, although not in the form of a venereal disease. Changes in social and environmental conditions triggered a change in symptoms and modes of transmission; the social and political disruptions of late-fifteenth-century Europe—widespread warfare, increased travel, changing sexual norms—account for the sudden and dramatic nature of the epidemic. The dispute about the origins of syphilis is unlikely to be settled any time soon, and, in any event, it is not my intention here to revisit this debate. What is clear, however, is that for Europeans living at the turn of the sixteenth century, syphilis constituted something new and horrifying.[90]

Perhaps a more relevant question for our purposes is: how did early modern Europeans themselves make sense of the sudden appearance of this horrible malady? The variety of names given the new disease offers an important clue. At stake in determining the origins of the disease, especially in one transmitted sexually, is the desire to attribute responsibility to a group other than one's own. New and bad diseases come from somewhere else, brought by people with bad habits. Thus, the Italians called it the French disease, a name that endured despite efforts by the French, who preferred to call it the disease of Naples. But nothing was so distant, foreign, and unknown than the New World and to many it came to seem natural that the new disease should have come from there. Not only did the sudden appearance of the French disease in Europe coincide with Columbus's voyages, but also one of the most popular early remedies came from America. A predominant belief of the day was that God always provided a corresponding cure in the same place that He inflicts a disease. This was guaiacum, sometimes called *palo santo*, a wood from a tree native to the West Indies. The wood was broken into very small pieces and boiled in water resulting in a decoction that was used both as a topical and internal medicine. Holy Wood's reputed miraculous effects were widely praised by patient and practitioners alike, and during the 1520s its use was adopted all over Europe. The treatment caused the patient to sweat profusely, a desirable effect according to humoral theory, as this rid the body of its impurities. Apart from its American provenance, guaiacum's popularity may also have been aided by its relatively mild side effects, especially when compared to the other standard treatment of the day, mercury, which caused horrendous suffering in its recipients. Although the topical and internal use of this drug was the only relatively effective means of treating syphilis for the next four hundred years, its overuse killed many patients by poisoning them.

ACHAQUES Y INDISPOSICIONES: EVERYDAY AILMENTS

Colonial documents suggest that an even broader experience of illness was formed by the less life-threatening physical ailments that tend to be overlooked by the historian. Minor maladies and discomforts—conditions that are routinely and successfully treated today—afflicted everyone and added to the general anxiety about health. Because contemporary conceptions of disease emphasized symptomology, people recognized that even minor symptoms could initiate a major decline. Health, as we will see later, was the product of a carefully preserved balance, not a state of permanency, thus the individual had every reason for closely observing changes in routine bodily functions and on the outer surfaces of the body. It is not surprising, then, that the concern with everyday health meant keeping a close watch on both the body's evacuations and cutaneous manifestations that now might be regarded as superficial.[91] Maladies that manifested themselves on the skin were one of the most common categories of everyday disorders; the manuals of domestic medicine are full of treatment advice for the boils, ulcers, sores, tumors, and swellings that afflicted everyone. Today, within the hierarchy of modern medicine, skin conditions are not considered serious threats to health, but in past centuries this was, in both theory and practice, a major area of concern.

An anonymous observer in sixteenth-century New Spain wrote that "the ordinary diseases of the Spanish are apostems from which they die."[92] As with fevers, these *apostemas*, or fluid-filled swellings, are another example of how early moderns named and treated symptoms as disease entities. And like fevers, too, apostems were a rather large and general diagnostic category. The surgeon Alonso López de Hinojosos, who wrote a practical handbook on surgery for the nonprofessional in 1578, devoted twenty-seven chapters to the various types of *apostemas*. Here he describes a bewildering variety of maladies from which people suffered: gangrene of the limbs or digits; carbuncles; *lamparones* (painful swellings of the neck); *empeines* (a pustular skin rash); *encordios* (swellings of the groin area); *sarna*, or scabies; and an infinite diversity of growths, bumps, and protuberances which tend to appear anywhere on the head, eyes, nostrils, ears, or on the breasts.[93] At one point during his travels through New Spain, Fray Alonoso Ponce was much indisposed by an apostem of his right nipple, which:

> . . . was growing each day and getting worse . . . and even though they made him many benefactions and they applied a thousand remedies, none of them helped, until they gave him a *piedra cornerina* [a type of stone], which had the virtue, once placed on the swelling, of sticking to the meat and sucking out, bit by bit, the bad humor and softening it and reducing the swelling a great deal . . .

Unfortunately, the padre comisario's *apostema* returned, along with other "*achaques e indisposiciones*" ("ailments and indispositions"), causing him several more months of agony.[94]

The continuous narration of miraculous cures that circulated through colonial Mexico contains an abundance of sufferers' testimony relating their experience with these kinds of ailments. Many examples can be found in painted ex-votos from the eighteenth century. The young child of Juan Pavón, a sacristan in Mexico City, was alleviated of "*apostema* in the throat" when he was anointed with lamp oil from the Virgin of Guadalupe's shrine. Don Juan de Peñafiel, a king's official, "desperate from *lamparones* and *empeines*," was cured when his skin was rubbed with the sacred dirt from the sanctuary of San Miguel. A young woman's illness produced "interior sores *(llagas ynteriores)* on the whole of her back so that she could not be in bed, seated or standing"; the pain was so severe it penetrated right through her "bones, nerves, and entrails, [so that] she was just waiting to die." Happily for this *doncella*, her suffering came to an end "after 19 days, without any remedy other than the image *(estampa)* of [San Miguel] that she had placed on her back." And, finally, there is the case of little Hipólito, the infant son of Spanish parents living in the city of Oaxaca, whose illness of "two *apostemas* right under the arms" required such extensive bandaging and binding that he "could not move for two days." The supplications to La Soledad, the patron saint of the city, were successful, but because the parents were slow in fulfilling their vow to commission the ex-voto, Hipólito suffered a relapse of "many symptoms [*accidentes*] all of them very mortal."[95] Apparently, the disease category of apostema was not limited to ailments that manifested themselves only on the surface of the body; internal organs were affected by apostems, too. A sixteenth-century resident of Mexico City writes to his wife in Seville about his desperate state of health: ". . . since coming here I have not had one day of health, and all of the month of July and August I was in bed, and without any hope, so that the doctors wanted to open me up, because they said that my disease was an apostem on my liver . . ." This letter-writer eventually got better—without surgery, luckily—but only after much bleeding and purging.[96]

Also prevalent and, judging from the bewildering variety of remedies offered to contemporaries, of crucial concern, was a whole host of conditions that were associated with urination, including the dreaded kidney stone. Afflictions associated with urination were a very common health problem. Contemporaries simply called this condition *mal de orina*, or disease of the urine, but the domestic medicine guides give some idea what this meant for the sufferer. Both Gregorio López and Esteyneffer describe these various problems as urine with blood, urine with rotten material, urination with pain, urination without sensation (incontinence), and inability to urinate. The infinite number of remedies for *mal de orina* also suggests that many people sought relief from these types of symptoms. Treatments ranged from the usual bleeding and purgings and the use of ordinary herbs and foods—*achiote* in chocolate, rose mallow, clover, sheep's milk, and recently laid chicken eggs—to more bizarre ingredients. López, for example, suggests that horse manure cooked in wine and placed hot on the patient's navel will help with blood in the urine; likewise, the sufferer of *orina podrida*, or urine with foul material, can be cured by drinking a mixture of rabbit's urine and *pulque blanco*.[97]

But surely the most dreaded malady associated with the urinary tract was *la piedra*, the kidney or bladder stone, a very common illness until the nineteenth century. Renal stones develop when abnormal concretions of calculi form in the kidneys or bladder, becoming impacted and sometimes obstructing the flow of urine. This condition, although not usually life-threatening, can cause its victim extreme discomfort and pain as the stones travel through the urinary tract. Stones originating in the bladder are rare today in industrialized countries, although they were quite common in earlier centuries; stones originating in the kidneys—"kidney stones"—today still affect about 5 percent of the population.[98] Poor nutrition and lack of variation in the diet—something that occurred at all levels of society—probably contributed to the prevalence of this condition in New Spain, as it did in Western Europe. That renal stones were a frequent health problem for many people is evident from the frequent references made to a vast assortment of remedies and practitioners that specialized in treating this malady. One study of Spanish medicine in the sixteenth and seventeenth centuries has identified a large group of practitioners whose activities were watched and debated in the Acts of the Castilian Court. These empirics were described as being proficient in the "art of extracting stones from the bladder and demolishing and curing those of the kidneys and curing growths and all pains of the urine (*pasiones de orina*), in men as well as women, without recourse to cutting with instruments (*hierros*), [in] boys and girls, and other aliments and illnesses that men tend to get in the scrotum and hidden parts . . ." The demand for these services must have been high as the royal authorities granted permission to many of these practitioners to teach their skills to others.[99]

Kidney stones were generally treated with medicines but sometimes more aggressive means were used to extract them. A doctor practicing in Mexico in the mid-sixteenth century witnessed an operation in which a stone "the size of an egg" was removed from a patient.[100] Lithotomy, the surgical removal of the stone, had been practiced from the first century AD by a method known as the "apparatus minor": a finger in the rectum forced the stone to bulge into the perineum, making it possible to cut and remove it without the use of other instruments. Early in the sixteenth century, a new method was widely adopted. Called the "apparatus major," it involved dilating and incising the urethra just in front of the bladder neck to allow the introduction of several instruments to extract the stone. This technique—which, in an age before anesthesia, must have been an excruciating experience for the patient—avoided damage to the prostate gland and seminal vesicles, which commonly led to excessive bleeding and even incontinence after the older technique. In the eighteenth century, new methods of stone extraction were developed and many surgeons promoted their own variations and instrumentation. Lithotomy, which had been practiced almost exclusively by unlicensed practitioners in the sixteenth century, was gradually appropriated by licensed surgeons by the end of the eighteenth.[101]

Eye disorders also were widespread, and of all the senses, the threat to sight caused the most anxiety. On one occasion, when her daughter was suffering from an eye inflammation, the Condesa de Miravalle sent mesquite wood, a common remedy for *mal de ojos*. Cataracts, or *nubes en los ojos*, were a common condition, the cause of which was usually attributed to the environment. According to compilers of the *Relaciones Geográficas* the Indians of Quautlatlauca suffered from them because they lived in a land that was "very white and dry," as did the residents of Tecpamatitlan, where the fog was so thick that "one can not see the houses, and besides causing sadness and melancholy, this is very damaging for the eyes, as many Indians in this village have cataracts."[102]

Another troublesome affliction was toothache. The surgeon López de Hinojosos's first piece of advice for this malady was "never let the barber pull a tooth until he has tried some remedies for the pain, like vinegar cooked with some pepper corns."[103] Tooth-pulling, performed by a barber-surgeon, or perhaps a more specialized *sacamuelas*, or "toothpuller," was almost always the treatment of last resort in an age before modern dentistry was able to treat tooth decay effectively. This does not mean, however, that people of past centuries did not pay attention to their dental health; in fact, lots of historical sources strongly indicate the contrary. Not only were they concerned with what to do about cavities, loose teeth, bleeding gums, abscesses, and, most important, ending the incessant pain of a decayed tooth, but they worried as well about how their teeth looked and breath smelled.[104] *La Gaceta de México*, a newspaper published in the later colonial years, is full of advertisements such as this one offering a "dental elixir which is very useful for the fluxuations and pains of the molars and teeth, roots and gums, it secures teeth firmly in place, gets rid of filth and tartar, and prevents scurvy and bad breath . . ." Included in the price of 10 reales was the exlir's own recipe, so one could reproduce the remedy at home.[105]

This exploration of everyday ailments could go on indefinitely. Even a casual glance at the remedies in circulation during the colonial period reveals a whole variety of other commonly endured conditions such as hernia, constipation, hemorrhoids, sciatica, rheumatism, and gout. In addition to these, women suffered from the usual menstrual problems, difficult pregnancies, dangerous deliveries, puerperal fever, *mal de madre*, and complications with breastfeeding. The ex-voto of Maria Narajo, painted in 1774, expresses, both pictorially and with text, the risky business that was childbirth at this time. ". . . around 9 in the evening Maria Naranjo began to have pains of childbirth and at dawn the next morning they had to remove the child by hand; the paturient continued to suffer with great risk to her life until [the next day]." Earnest appeals were made by the family and midwife to Nuesta Señora de Tulantongo, to whom the ex-voto is dedicated.[106] Nor can we overlook the early modern preoccupation with mood and state of mind. In his chapter on melancholia, Farfán notes that this surprisingly common disease afflicts and torments many, and that men and women scarcely reach the age of twenty when they begin to complain of it. Some of the symptoms include generalized "fears and frights," abnormal fears of death, insomnia, lack of appetite, and a "tightening of the throat and a feeling like one is being drowned," the latter that sounds very much like the "panic attack" of today. True to his Galenic training, Farfán explained this disease in terms of physical factors. One form of melancholia arises from "sediments" of the blood, and is cold and dry, whereas another originates in the liver and "burns with excessive heat."[107] The Condesa de Miravalle's chronically ailing daughter, Maria Antonia, appears to have suffered greatly from this disorder. In one letter the mother warns her daughter to be mindful of her moods "because from these *melancolicas* come many bad things."[108]

And, finally, to these endemic and chronic illnesses must be added the dangers of everyday life. Falls from buildings and scaffolding, fires, drownings, mishaps with tools, overturned carriages, falls and kicks from horses and mules, and encounters with bandits were just some of the hazards people encountered. The personal testimonies in the form of ex-votos left by survivors of these accidents provide one of the best windows we have to view this side of life. A man is thrown from his mule and has trouble getting clear of the bucking animal; another is attacked by thieves on the road to his house, stabbed in the side, and left for dead. A third, as shown in this ex-voto from the eighteenth century, takes a bad fall while he is collecting corn from a storage area on a rooftop.[109] In these personal testimonies from the eighteenth century, the victims miraculously survived their ordeals. But in an age without adequate emergency services, the trauma from accidents and violence must have been especially feared as blood loss could quickly kill. The maintenance of health and the relief of anxiety about health thus created a high demand for all kinds of medical advice and care.

NOTES

1. Jared Diamond, *Guns, Germs, and Steel: The Fates of Human Societies* (New York: W.W. Norton & Co., 1999).

2. Robert McCaa, "The Peopling of Mexico from Origins to Revolution," in *A Population History of North America*, ed. Michael R. Haines and Richard H. Steckel (Cambridge: Cambridge University Press, 2000) pp. 248–9; Rebecca Storey, *Life and Death in the Ancient City of Teotihuacan: A Modern Paleodemographic Synthesis* (Tuscaloosa: University of Alabama Press, 1992), p. 237.

3. Sherburn Cook, "The Incidence and Significance of Disease among the Aztecs and Related Tribes," *The Hispanic American Historical Review*, 26 (1946), 332; Carlos Viesca T. "Hambruna y epidemia en Anáhuac (1450–1454) en la época de Moctezuma Illhuicamina," in *Ensayos sobre la historia de las epidemias en México*, ed. Enrique Florescano and Elsa Malvido (México: Instituto Méxicano del Seguro Social, 1982), p. 163.

4. Marshall T. Newman, "Aboriginal New World Epidemilogy and Medical Care, and the Impact of Old World Disease Imports," *Physical Anthropology*, 45:3 (November 1976), 667–72; Lourdes Márques Morfín, et al., "Health and Nutrition in Prehispanic Mesoamerica," in *The Backbone of History: Health and Nutrition in the Western Hemisphere*, ed. Richard H. Steckel and Jerome C. Rose (Cambridge University Press, 2002); Robert McCaa, "The Peopling of Mexico"; Rebecca Storey, *Life and Death in the Ancient City of Teotihuacan*; Lourdes Márqiez Morfín, et al., *Playa del Carmen: Una población de la costa oriental en el postclásico (un estudio osteológico)* (México: Instituto Nacional de Antropología e Historia, 1982).

5. Storey, p. 18; Douglas H. Ubelaker, "Patterns of Disease in Early North American Populations," in Haines and Steckel, p. 55.

6. Mark Nathan Cohen, *Health and the Rise of Civilization* (New Haven, CT: Yale University Press, 1989); T. Aiden Cockburn, "Infectious Disease in Ancient Populations," *Current Anthropology*, 12 (1971), 45–66.

7. Márquez Morfín, et al., "Health and Nutrition," p. 15; Storey, p. 231.

8. Storey, p. 257.

9. MaCaa, "The Peopling of Mexico," pp. 246–7.

10. Márquez Morfín, et al., "Health and Nurtrition," pp. 20–1; on tortilla making and women, see Arnold Bauer, "Millers and Grinders: Technology and Household Economy in Meso-America," *Agricultural History*, 64:1 (Winter 1990), 1–17.

11. Márques Morfín, et al., "Health and Nutrition," p. 23.

12. Ubelaker, pp. 57–63; MaCaa, "The Peopling of Mexico," p. 246.

13. Fray Bernardino de Sahagún, *Florentine Codex, General History of the Things of New Spain*, ed. and trans. C. E. Dibble and A. J. O. Anderson, 12 books (Salt Lake City: University of Utah Press, 1950–69), I:31, XI:173; Bernard R. Ortiz de Montellano, *Aztec Medicine, Health, and Nutrition* (New Brunswick, NJ: Rutgers University Press, 1990), p. 120.

14. Newman, p. 669; Cook, "Disease among the Aztecs," pp. 325–7.

15. Alfred Crosby Jr., *The Colombian Exchange: Biological and Cultural Consequences of 1442* (Westport, CT: Greenwood Press, 1972), p. 37.

16. Margaret Pelling, *The Common Lot: Sickness, Medical Occupations and the Urban Poor in Early Modern England* (London: Longman, 1998), p. 28.

17. Zaida M. Feliciano, "Mexico's Demographic Transformation: 1920 to 1990," in Haines and Steckel, p. 608.

18. Kenneth F. Kiple, "The Ecology of Disease," in *Companion Encyclopedia of the History of Medicine*, 2 vols., ed. W. F. Bynum and Roy Porter (London: Routledge, 1993), Vol. I, pp. 375–7, hereafter cited as CEHM.

19. Diamond, p. 210.

20. Enrique Florescano and Elsa Malvido, *Ensayos sobre la historia de las epidemias México*; Alfed W. Crosby Jr., "Conquistador y pestilencia: The First New World Pandemic and the Fall of the Great Indian Empires," *HAHR*, 47 (1967), 321–37; Alfred W. Crosby Jr., *The Columbian Exchange: Biological and Cultural Consequences of 1492*; Robert McCaa, "Spanish and Nahuatl Views on Smallpox and Demographic Catastrophe in Mexico," *Journal of Interdisciplinary History*, XXV:3 (Winter 1995), 397–431; Noble David Cook and W. George Lovell, *Secret Judgements of God: Old World Disease in Colonial Spanish America* (Norman: University of Oklahoma Press, 1991); Thomas M. Whitmore, *Disease and Death in Early Colonial Mexico: Simulating Amerindian Depopulation* (Boulder, CO: Westview Press, 1992).

21. Cook and Lovell, "Unraveling the Web of Disease," in *Secret Judgements of God*, p. 216; Sherburne F. Cook and Woodrow Borah, *The Indian Population of Central Mexico, 1531–1610*, Ibero-Americana, 44 (Berkeley and Los Angeles, 1960); Shelburn F. Cook and Woodrow Borah, *Essays in Population History*, 3 vols. (Berkeley and Los Angeles: University of California Press, 1971–9).

22. Whitmore, pp. 109–20.

23. Charles Gibson, *The Aztecs under Spanish Rule: A History of the Indians of the Valley of Mexico, 1519–1810* (Stanford: Stanford University Press, 1964), pp. 448–9; Peter Gerhard, *A Guide to the Historical Geography of New Spain*, rev. ed. (Norman: University of Oklahoma Press, 1993), p. 23.

24. Anthony Pagden, ed. and trans., *Hernán Cortés: Letters from Mexico* (New Haven, CT: Yale University Press, 1986), pp. 164–5; Bernal Diaz del Castillo, *Historia verdadera de la conquista de la Nueva España* (México: Alianza Editorial, 1991), p. 416; *Anals de Tenochtitlan* (Codex Aubin) in *We People Here: Nahuatl Accounts of the Conquest of Mexico*, ed. and trans. James Lockhart (Berkeley: University of California Press, 1993), p. 279.

25. Book Twelve of *The Florentine Codex*, in Lockhart, *We People Here*, pp. 181–5.

26. Crosby, *The Columbian Exchange*, p. 46; *Cecil Textbook of Medicine, 19th ed.*, ed. James B. Wyngaarden, M.D., Lloyd H. Smith Jr., M.D., and J. Claude Bennett, M.D. (Philadelphia: W.B. Saunders Company, 1992), pp. 1842–3; Lovell and Cook, "Unraveling the Web of Disease," p. 218; Richard Preston, "The Demon in the Freezer: How Smallpox, A Disease Officially Eradicated Twenty Years Ago, became the Biggest Threat We Now Face," *The New Yorker*, July 12, 1999, pp. 44–64.

27. Toribio de Benavente o Motolinía, *Memoriales o libro de las cosas de la Nueva España y de los naturales de ella*, ed. Edmundo O'Gorman (México: UNAM, 1971), p. 21; Licenciado Lucas Vásquez de Ayllón, "Relación que hizo el Licenciado Lucas Vásquez de Ayllón, de sus diligencias para estorbar el rompiemiento entre Cortés y Narváez," in *Cartas y relaciones de Hernán Cortés al Emperador Carlos V*, ed. Pascual de Gayango (Paris, 1866), p. 42, quoted in McCaa, "Spanish and Nahuatl Views on Smallpox," p. 432.

28. Crosby, *Ecological Imperialism: The Biological Expansion of Europe, 900–1900*, (Cambridge: Cambridge University Press, 1986), p. 286; Hanns J. Prem, "Disease Outbreaks in Central Mexico during the Sixteenth Century," in Cook and Lovell, p. 25.

29. Kiple, pp. 368–9; Crosby, *Ecological Imperialism*, p. 34.

30. Kiple, pp. 358–9; Diamond, pp. 203–5.

31. Diamond, pp. 202–3.

32. Ibid., pp. 212–13; Crosby, *Ecological Imperialism*, pp. 30–1.

33. Diamond, p. 213.

34. Motolinía, p. 413; "Carta del virey de la Nueva España, Don Martín Enriquez al Rey Don Felipe II," in *Cartas de Indias* (Madrid, 1877), Vol. I, p. 331; "Carta de Fray Domingo de Betanzos," in *Colección de documentos para la historia de México*, ed. Joaquín García Icazbalceta (México, 1866), p. 200; Diego Muñoz Camargo, "Descripción de la ciudad y provincia de Tlaxcala," in *Relaciones Geográficas del siglo XVI: Tlaxcacla*, ed. René Acuña, 10 vols. (Méxcio: UNAM, 1984), Vol. V., pp. 75–6, hereafter cited as RG.

35. Sahagún, cited in German Somolinos d'Ardpos, "Las epidemias en México durante el siglo XVI," Florescano and Malvido, p. 208.

36. Eloise Quiñones Keber, *Codex Tellerianso-Remensis: Rituals, Divination, and History in a Pictorial Aztec Manuscript* (Austin: University of Texas Press, 1995), Folio 46v, pp. 96 and 238.

37. *Papeles de Nueva España publicados de orden y con fondos del gobierno mexicano por Francisco del Paso y Troncoso*, 2a serie, *Geográfica y Estadística* (México: Editoral Cosmos, 1979): *Relación de Cuauhquilpan*, p. 307; *Relación de Huezutla*, p. 185; *Relación de Mexicalzinco*, p. 195: *Relación de Ocopetlayuca*, p. 258; *Relación de Atitalaquia*, p. 202, hereafter cited as PNE.

38. Ciudad Real, Antonio de, *Tratado curioso y docto de las grandezas de la Nueva España*, (México: Instituto de Investigaciones Históricas, UNAM, 1993) Vol. II, p.131.

39. Motolinía, p. 21.

40. "Juan López de Soria a la condesa de Ribadavia," México: November 30, 1576, in Enrique Otte, editor, *Cartas Privadas de Emigrantes a Indias, 1540–1616* (México: Fondo de Cultura Económica, 1993), pp. 96–7.

41. Hans Zinsser, *Rats, Lice, and History*, (Boston: Atlantic Monthly Press, 1963) p. 120; Whitmore, p. 54.

42. Cited in Gibson, p. 449.

43. Prem, p. 33.

44. Fray Gerónimo de Mendieta, *Historia Eclesiástica Indiana* (México: Editorial Salvador Chavez Hayhoe, 1945), Vol. III, p.174.

45. *Códice de 1576*, cited in Somolinos, 1982, pp. 212–13.

46. PNE: "Relación de Ocopetlayuca," p. 258; Gerhard, p. 329.

47. Francisco Javier Alegre, *Historia de la Compania de Jesús en Nueva España*, ed. Carlos María Bustamante (México, 1841–2), Vol. II, p. 262; see also Cayetano de Cabrerra y Quintero, *Escudo de Armas de México* (México: Instituto Mexicano del Seguro Social, 1981); América Molina del Villar, *La Nueva España y el matlazahuatl, 1736–1739* (México: Centro de Investigaciones y Estudios Superiores en Antropología Social/El Colegio de Michoacán, A.C., 2001).

48. Zinsser, pp. 216–64; Nicholás León, "Qué era el Matlazáhuatl y qué el Cocoliztli en los tiempos precolumbinos y en la época hispana?" in Florescano and Malvino, Vol. II, p. 383; Cook and Lovell, "Unraveling the Web of Disease," pp. 225–7.

49. Francisco de las Barras y Aragón, "Viaje del astrónomo francés Chappe a California en 1796, y noticias de J. A. Alzate sobre la historia natural de Nueva España,"*Anuario de estudios americanos*, Vol. I (1944), p. 767, cited in Donald B. Cooper, *Epidemic Disease in Mexico City, 1761–1813: An Administrative, Social, and Medical Study* (Austin: University of Texas Press, 1965), p. 49.

50. Cooper, p. 54.

51. Ex-voto to Our Lady of Sorrows and to San Sebastian. Anonymous, 1761. Franz Mayer Museum, Mexico City.

52. Archivo Manuel Romero de Terreros (Pachuca, Mexico): *Miravalles*, 23 de Mayo, 1762; 27 de enero, 1763; and 12 de noviembree, 1761, hereafter cited as AMRT.

53. Elsa Malvido, "Cronología de epidemias y crisis agrícolas en la época colonial," and "Efectos de las epidemias y hambrunas en la población de México (1519–1810)," in Florescano and Malvido, pp. 171–8, 179–200.

54. Cabrera y Quintero, pp. 67–71; Gibson, pp. 448–51; MaCaa, "The Peopling of Mexico," p. 260.

55. MaCaa, "The Peopling of Mexico," p. 260.

56. Ciudad Real, Vol. I, p. 149; RG, I: 30, V: 38, 74 346, 408, VI: 79, 88, 302; *PNE*, pp. 10, 76, 91, 103, 120, 287; AMRT, *Miravalles*, 2 de julio de 1757.

57. Juan de Cárdenas, *Primera parte de los problemas y secretos maravillosos de las Indias* (Madrid: Alianza Editorial, 1988), pp. 240–1.

58. Fray Agustín Farfán, *Tractado breve de medicina*, facs. ed. (Madrid: Ediciones Culturas Hispanica, 1944), pp. 1–2.

59. Ibid., p. 2.

60. "Alonso de Alcocer a su hermano Juan de Colonia, en Madrid," México: 10 de diciembre, 1577; "Gaspar de Vargas a Alonso Pérez Pocasangre, in Jaén," México: 5 de noviembre, 1564; "Maria Diaz a su hija Inés Díaz, en Sevilla,"México: 31.de marzo, 1577, in Otte, pp. 98–9, 45, 97–8.

61. Farfán, pp. 9–10; Esteyneffer, pp. 272–3.

62. "Juan de Brihuega a su hermano Pedro Garcia, en Briguega," Puebla: 16 de enero, 1572, in Otte, p. 154.

63. RG, II: 154, 168.

64. "Marcos Ortiz a su padre," México: 22 de febrero, 1569, in Otte, p.54; Ciudad Real, I. p. 26.

65. Lenard G. Wilson, "Fevers," in CEHM, pp. 384–5.

66. Cook, "Disease among the Aztecs and Related Tribes," p. 323; Ortiz de Montellano, p, 122.

67. Miguel E. Bustamante, "La fiebre amarilla en México y su origen en América," in Florescano and Malvido, p. 27; Andrew L. Knaut. "Yellow Fever and the Late Colonial Public Health Response in the Port of Veracruz," *HAHR*, 77:4 (Nov. 1997), 623. For nineteenth-century travelers' accounts, see Salvador Novo, *Breve historia y antología sobre la fiebre amarilla* (México: Secretaría de Salubridad y Asistencia, 1964).

68. Francisco Ajofrín, *Diario del viaje que . . . hizo a la América en el siglo XVIII el P. Fray Francisco Ajofrín Capuchino*, 2 vols. (Madrid:Archivo Documental Espanol, 1958), Vol. I, p. 37.

69. Knaut, pp. 623–4.

70. James S. Ward, *Yellow Fever in Latin America: A Geographical Study* (Liverpool: Center for Latin American Studies—University of Liverpool, 1972), p. 18.

71. Knaut, p. 627.

72. *Ibid.*, pp. 622, 626–7; on the Spanish American fleet system, see Peter Bakewell, *A History of Latin America: Empires and Sequels, 1450–1930* (Oxford: Blackwell Publishers, 1997), pp. 199–200.

73. Ward, p. 15.

74. Lourdes Márquez Morfín, *Sociedad colonial y enfermedad: Un ensayo de osteopathología diferencial* (México: Instituto Nacional de Anthropología e Historia, 1980), pp. 79–81, 99–100.

75. R. E. Hughes, "Scurvy," in *The Cambridge World History of Food*, 2 vols., ed. Kenneth F. Kiple and Kriemhild Coneè Ornelas (Cambridge: Cambridge University Press, 2000), Vol. I, pp. 988–9.

76. Henry R. Wagner *Spanish Voyages to the Northwest Coast of America in the Sixteenth Century* (San Francisco: California Historical Society, 1929), pp. 245–6, 260.

77. Margaret Pelling, *The Common Lot: Sickness, Medical Occupations and the Urban Poor in Early Modern England* (London: Longman, 1998), p. 28.

78. *Gaceta de México*, "Engargos,"martes 10 de julio de 1787, Vol. II, no. 38, p. 384; "Engargos," jueves 12 de noviembre de 1795, Vol. III, no. 57, p. 498.

79. Joaquín García Icazbalceta, *Bibliografía mexicana del siglo XVI* (México: Fondo de Cultura Economica, 1954), p. 227.

80. Josefina Muriel, *Hospitales de la Nueva España* (México: UNAM, 1990), Vol. I, p. 160.

81. Cárdenas, pp. 221–2.

82. Aria de Benavides, *Secretos de cirugía*, p. 66.

83. Bernal Díaz, p. 262.

84. Wesley W. Spink, M.D., *Infectious Diseases: Prevention and Treatment in the Nineteenth and Twentieth Centuries* (Minneapolis: University of Minnesota Press, 1978), pp. 305–6.

85. J. D. Oriel, *The Scars of Venus: A History of Venereology* (London: Springer-Verlag, 1994), pp. 35–41.

86. Crosby, *The Columbian Exchange*, pp. 124–5; Jon Arrizabalaga, John Henderson, and Roger French, *The Great Pox: The French Disease in Renaissance Europe* (New Haven, CT: Yale University Press, 1997), pp. 25–6.

87. Allan M. Brandt, "Sexually Transmitted Diseases," in CEHM, Vol. I, pp. 566–7; Esteyneffer, Vol. I, p. 346.

88. Crosby, *The Columbian Exchange*, p. 123.

89. Oriel, p. 11.

90. Crosby, *The Columbian Exchange*, pp. 122–47; Allan M. Brandt, "Sexually Transmitted Diseases," in CEHM, Vol. I, pp. 562–5.

91. Margaret Pelling, *The Common Lot: Sickness*, p. 204.

92. Francisco del Paso y Toncoso, ed., *Epistolario de Nueva España, 1505–1818*, Vol. XV (México: José Porrúa e Hijos, 1940), p. 59.

93. Alonoso López de Hinojosos, *Suma y recopilación de curugia con un arte para sangrar muy útil y provechosa* (México: Academia Nacional de Medicina, 1977).

94. Ciudad Real, Vol. I, pp. 43, 45–7.

95. *Dones y promesas*, pp. 67 (cat. 69), 51 (cat. 104), 57 (cat. 83); Hipólito's ex-voto, 1743: Museo de la Soledad, Oaxaca, Mexico.

96. "Hernán Ruiz a su mujer Mariana de Montedoca en Sevilla," México: Oct. 21, 1584 in Otte, p. 108–9.

97. López, pp. 274–6; Esteyneffer, pp. 407–18; "achiote en chocoate" in Ciudad Real, Vol. I, p. 241.

98. *Cecil Textbook of Medicine*, pp. 603–8.

99. Rafael Muñoz Garrido, "Empiricos sanitarios españoles de los siglos XVI y XVII," *Cuadernos de historia de la medicina española*, Vol. 6, 1967, pp. 101–33, esp. p. 102.

100. Garcia Icazbalceta, *Bibliografía mexicana* p. 228.

101. Ghislaine Lawrence, "Surgery (Traditonal)," in CEHM, Vol. II, p. 979.

102. AMRT *Miravalles*, 9 de enero, 1760; RG:V, p. 210; Ciudad Real, Vol. II, p. 18.

103. López de Hinojosos, p. 104.

104. Esteyneffer, pp. 235–42.

105. *Gaceta de México*, "Engargos," martes 27 de mayor de 1788, Vol. III, no. 9, p. 72.

106. Ex-voto to Our Lady of Tulantongo. Anonymous, 1774. Collection of María and Gonzalo Méndez, Mexico City, Mexico.

107. Farfán, pp. 107–13.

108. AMRT *Miravalles*, 24 de junio de 1762.

109. Ex-votos from the Museo de la Soledad, Oaxaca: Joseph Antonio de los Angeles, 10 de junio de 1746; don Francisco Valencia, 26 de enero de 1762; Julian Castellanos, 21 de noveimbre de 1767.

2. DOCTORS, BLEEDERS, AND VIRGINS

The origins of a medical marketplace lie in the sufferer's attempt to find an explanation for his or her disorder and a means to restore health. Indeed, one might argue that the search for relief constitutes the historical basis for the healer's unique social role. As human populations developed more complex social systems, medical expertise became the vocation of particular individuals with specialized knowledge. Although domestic medicine remained the first line of defense against disease, it was often augmented by "medicine men, diviners, witchsmellers, and shamans, and in due course, by herbalists, birth-attendants, bone-setters, barber-surgeons and healer-priests." Social complexity created opportunities for enterprising practitioners to peddle their goods and skills as demand for medicines grew and new forms of healing evolved. Moreover, the need to rationalize and theorize sickness became greater as patients demanded that healers put a name to their pain and suffering. In other words, the rise of complex societies created the right conditions for the growth of medicine as a belief system and an occupation.[1] Leaving the belief system of medicine to the following two chapters, the present one continues to look at the day-to-day reality of sufferers, this time with a focus on the types of medical services that were available to them, first in Postclassic Mesoamerica, and then in the colonial world of New Spain.

What did people of past centuries do when they became ill? Drawing on a variety of systems, their responses to sickness were diverse and their choices were dictated by such factors as perceived seriousness of illness, cost and availability of care, distance from medical expertise, and past experience. Most people, at least in the initial stages of an illness, relied on the time-honored art of domestic medicine. The first level at which sickness is recognized, defined, and treated is at home, in consultation with family members, close friends, and neighbors. Although the role of domestic healing has diminished greatly with the professionalization of medicine in the twentieth century, in earlier times it constituted the bulk of health care, for even when outside advice and treatment were sought, the nursing of the patient usually took place at home. The primary providers of this health care were, most likely, local women—wives, mothers, grandmothers, daughters, and friends—all sharing in a basic knowledge of common ailments and popular remedies. Through the centuries, the basic repertoire of domestic medicine has always included of a hodgepodge of empirical and supernatural measures: special brews made from plants or animal parts, changes in diet, the use of charms, talismans, prayers, and special rituals. Only when illness was deemed too complex for lay understanding was expertise sought outside the home.

The art and actual day-to-day practice of medicine in the early modern period was very broad and heterogeneous, especially if we compare it to our own time. Today, at least in Western societies in which professional medicine is more narrowly defined, care for the sick is provided by a relatively small range of medical institutions and practitioners who are similarly trained and socially homogeneous. In contrast, the medical marketplace in an early modern society such as colonial Mexico consisted of a diverse assortment of secular and religious healers. The familiar tripartite hierarchy of professionals—the physicians, surgeons, and apothecaries—who were trained in rational Galenic theories, practiced alongside an array of irregular and popular healers who worked within a vigorous and evolving system of traditional medicine: bonesetters, barbers, itinerant tooth-pullers, oculists, *sacadores de la piedra*, midwives, curanderos, witches, *titici* ("indigenous doctors"), nurses, priests, and nuns. Any view of medical practice as it really was in colonial Mexico must include all practitioners involved with dispensing care. Throughout this study, therefore, my definition of a "medical practitioner" includes anyone who was engaged in caring for the sick, anyone who appeared to sufferers themselves as medically skilled and experienced. The distinction that separates popular from sanctioned healers was less relevant to contemporaries than we moderns imagine; whether a healer was legitimate or not was often a question of licensing and lay in the eyes of the beholder. Charges of quackery more generally came from contemporary professional groups. Much of the surviving historical record regarding medical practice in New Spain was generated by licensed practitioners in their efforts to check the proliferation of unlicensed empirics, also known as *intrusos*, for their "intrusion" into a supposedly controlled field of medicine. This is not to say that unethical practices did not abound; they undoubtedly did, but opportunities for ethical misconduct existed at all levels. It is important, therefore, not to allow "the special pleading of contemporary pressure groups to lead the historian into undervaluing the activities of arbitrarily defined sections of the medical community."[2]

That the early modern medical landscape was such a diverse place is understandable when we consider the varied forms of contemporary medicine. For one thing, most people believed, in varying degrees, that the causes and cures of disease emanated from both the natural and supernatural world. This led to a proliferation of healing strategies and the specialists who hawked them. Many healers, especially those who viewed medicine through its Hippocratic lens, treated patients primarily using the physical properties of natural substances—plants, foods, and animal parts—along with time-honored therapies such as bleeding and purging. Others promoted their unique knowledge of the destructive and restorative actions of divine entities, tapping into supernatural zones through incantations, charms, offerings, and hallucinogenic drugs. In practice, most practitioners combined the elements of rational and divine medicine; university-trained doctors acknowledged the powerful role played by divine providence in any illness, whereas indigenous healers almost always included physical remedies in treating their patients—the use of tobacco, for example, was common, as was bathing and purging. In addition to the flesh-and-blood healers on the ground, a cult of saints as healers flourished throughout New Spain, generating a hierarchy of spiritual figures who specialized in miracle cures for certain ailments. Commonly, these divine members of the medical marketplace—the virgins and Christ figures that became important locally, and some, such as the Virgin of Guadalupe, throughout the viceroyalty—were the last to be appealed to in the "hierarchy of resort," an indication of desperation when other earthly measures had failed.

Diversity in the medical marketplace also must have been invigorated by the limited efficacy of contemporary therapies. Because no single group of practitioners could reliably cure better than another, people tended to shop around. The domain of medical knowledge, especially in the sixteenth and seventeenth centuries, had not yet fused into the two distinct spheres that would later emerge in the nineteenth and twentieth centuries: the scientific, print-culture knowledge of the educated and, later, the highly specialized professional, in contrast to the traditional, oral-based folk medicine of the lower orders. Rather, multiple modes of medicine existed simultaneously, overlapping and competing for authority. Although one might be hard pressed to characterize this as a pluralistic arena of medical discourse, medical information did flow across divisions of class and gender. The exchange of medical advice up and down the social ladder makes sense in an age when the threat of disease, disability, and death was felt by all. In her work on sixteenth-century England, Margaret Pelling has written that the perils to life and limb were not equally shared by all groups but enough so to bridge social divisions and to create something like a "common sense of human frailty."

> Such fears, it should be stressed, were leveling without being democratic. Social barriers remained intact, but networks of information about cures and practitioners ramified across divisions of gender, age, and class. When it came to illness, a Privy Councilor could learn from his laundress, a husband from his wife, a philosopher from an old woman, a gentleman from his servant, . . . This did not imply real or lasting tolerance, nor would one party to the exchange of information necessarily refrain from taking advantage of the other. However, something about the imperative to communicate on such matters was recognized by all parties, and proved a major obstacle to attempts by medical corporations at restriction and regulation.[3]

Just as in early modern England, the menace of disease in colonial Mexico stimulated all sorts of activity to counter sickness. Its medical marketplace was a multifarious and intricate place, so it is difficult to untangle its layers, especially over a distance of many centuries, but some general observations should be kept in mind as we survey the medical landscape of New Spain. The polarities we tend to look for in more modern medical systems—professional versus lay, literate versus oral, secular versus religious—did not begin to form in Mexico until the late colonial period, and only then in urban areas. This is not to say that competing systems did not exist. They did, but the boundaries between them were much more fluid than we would find today between, say, faith healing and biomedicine.

In this chapter, I set out to describe the variety of healers that comprised the medical marketplace in New Spain. Because native Mexicans—the largest segment of the population until the last part of the colonial period—bring their own distinct healing traditions into the mosaic of colonial practices, I begin with a brief look at what historical sources tell us about medical practitioners before the conquest. For New Spain, I turn, first, to the familiar tripartite of formally educated medical professionals: the doctors, surgeons, and pharmacists—distinct categories that don't hold up in the day-to-day reality of a severe shortage of such practitioners on the ground. The majority of the population received primary care not from formally trained and licensed physicians, but from our next large, and rather amorphous, group: the barber-surgeons, midwives, and curanderos—empirically trained, and practically all of whom practiced outside the law. The chapter ends with a focus on the Church's role in providing medical care and solace through the establishment of hospitals and the promotion of a cult of saints with miraculous healing powers.

HEALERS IN MESOAMERICA

Scholars of Mesoamerican culture have been more successful in identifying the basic ideas that underlay Nahua medicine than they have been in learning about its actual day-to-day practice. This failing is one of historical sources, not scholarship. With very few exceptions, everything we know today about ancient Mexican medicine comes from documents that were compiled by Spaniards after the fall of Tenochtitlan in 1521. The discovery of the New World aroused an enormous amount of interest in Europe; the accounts of fact-finding expeditions were mixed with fantastical stories of monsters, savages, and mythical animals. Of particular interest were reports of American medicinal plants and substances, stimulating European chroniclers to compile herbals of the new materials. In New Spain, the two major works of this sort, Francisco Hernández's *Historia Natural de la Nueva España* and Martín de la Cruz's *Badianus Codex*, stand alongside Fray Bernardino de Sahagun's encyclopedic work on preconquest life as the major sources on Mesoamerican medicine.[4] The shortcomings of these texts as historical records—for example, the way the authors filtered native medicine through their own European medical concepts, or the way in which Sahagún cleansed much of his informants' information of its supernatural content—have already been discussed extensively by the many scholars who have used them. But it is worth reiterating the point here about how little interest Europeans actually had in the native practice of medicine; their interest lay almost exclusively in the medicines of the Americas and how they could be incorporated into a European medical complex. Consequently, the chroniclers are mostly silent on the native dispensers of these drugs. The healing strategies of native doctors mingled the sacred with the rational much more extensively than anything with which European authorities were comfortable; therefore, much of the interest in them was limited to recognizing and extirpating the idolatry in their practices. Hernando Ruiz de Alarcón's *Treatise on Superstitions*, written in the early seventeenth century specifically for this purpose, gives us some idea of what native healers were doing a hundred years after the conquest, but because he is exclusively concerned with eradicating paganism, his exposition of Nahua medicine tends to overlook empirical techniques, centering his attention, and scorn, on the "superstitious" incantations used by indigenous curanderos.[5]

The most thorough colonial source from which scholars have assembled their impressions about Mesoamerican medicine, indeed about all aspects of pre-Columbian life, is the work of Sahagún. The *Florentine Codex* and its Spanish version, the *Historia general de las cosas de Nueva España*, contain two types of information about medicine.[6] In the sections in which Sahagún specifically intended to document Nahua medical knowledge, the information appears to be more deliberately self-censored than in other sections. Here the connections between illness and religion were deemphasized or left out entirely, leaving the impression of less supernatural involvement in Nahua medicine than there was in reality. But in other sections of the work, the answers to questions on different subjects spontaneously reveal information about the effects deities and those who manipulated magic had on health and illness, making it possible for scholars to cross-check and correlate them in order to flesh out more complex, holistic medical concepts and practices.[7] It is also from these sections that our sketchy notions of Mesoamerican healers—who they were, what services they offered, and where they fit into the social landscape—are derived.

In the highly evolved society of Postclassic central Mexico, the *tícitl* (*titici*, plural), a Náhuatl word we might loosely translate as "doctor," or "someone skilled in the art of curing," was no simple healer, at least in Western conceptions of that word. His function was a complex one in which he was required to apply his ample knowledge of the physical world in accordance with his understanding of the gods and the manner in which they intervened into human affairs.[8] The medicine of the Nahuas was much more entangled with religion than the medical knowledge emerging from medieval and early modern universities in Europe. Consequently, the *tícitl*'s role combined sacerdotal functions with hands-on, empirically based therapy. Anthropologists have long argued that the tight link between religion and medicine—something found in most cultures throughout history—originates from the collective and personal anxiety humans experience as they face the threat of suffering and death that illness brings. For the Nahuas, this vulnerability was magnified by a sense of personal dependency nurtured in the rigid social structure created under Mexica rule. According to Aguirre Beltrán, each individual in this highly militaristic society was "subjected, from the first years of life, to rigorous disciplines which had the tendency to create in his [or her] personality a constellation of [behavior patterns based on the notions of] disobedience-punishment, obedience-gratification." These notions permeated all aspects of life, including medicine.[9] Thus punishment from any number of deities that populated the Mesoamerican universe often came in the form of illness. But the etiological beliefs of the Nahuas, a topic we explore in depth in Chapter 4, were not so simplistic, attributing all ailments to gods angry with human failings. Rather, the origins of illness were quite complex, including and often intertwining two types of causes:

> those that we would call natural—excesses, accidents, deficiencies, exposure to sudden temperature changes, contagions, and the like—and those caused by the intervention of nonhuman beings or of human beings with more than normal powers. For example, a native could think that his rheumatic problems came from the supreme will of Titlacahuan, from the punishment sent by Tlaloque for not having performed a certain rite, from direct attack by a being who inhabited a certain spring, and from prolonged chilling in cold water; the native would not consider it all as a confluence of diverse causes but as a complex.[10]

The extent of the *tícitl's* expertise, then, reached way beyond the parameters of medicine understood in the Western sense.

Just what were the tasks of the *tícitl*? The native physicians informing Sahagún tell us that a good doctor is one that is "well informed, a good judge of the properties of herbs, stones, trees, and roots, someone experienced in cures." He also had to be proficient in the art of "setting bones, purging, bleeding and cupping, and closing wounds." Yet when Sahagún tells us that a bad doctor is one that "uses sorcery and superstitions in order to know how to make good cures," he is also describing a set of skills that every good physician in Mesoamerica would have had.[11] In fact, the medical knowledge of a competent *tícitl* would have been quite extensive, spanning both the supernatural and physical worlds. He would need to know, for instance, when and how individual gods provoke and cure disease; the inner workings of witchcraft and how to counteract its damaging effects; the functions of *tonalli* (an important animistic entity located in the head) and the effects of its loss on the body; the specific symptoms of numerous diseases; the properties of a myriad of medicines, and knowledge of the plants, animals, or minerals they come from, including where, when, and in what conditions to collect them and how to prepare them; and finally, be able to perform the essential rituals necessary for curing the sick.[12] Diagnosis consisted of identifying, first, where the illness was located in the patient's body, and, second, its cause. This process, by its nature, involved prognostication, a procedure that, although an essential component to medicine for the indigenous practitioner and patient alike, was later labeled superstitious by European witnesses. "By this fortune-telling they determine what the cause of illness may be, what the medicine will be, or whether none will be of any help."[13] The knotting and unknotting of cords, looking for signs in the water, the tossing of maize kernels, the measuring of the left forearm with the right palm, and the ingestion of hallucinogenics, such as *peyote* or *ololiuhqui* were all important tools in the process of diagnosis and prognosis.[14] Combined with special incantations and orations these types of actions employed throughout the therapeutic process were the standard ways in which the *tícitl* worked.

The field of medicine was open to Nahuas of both genders. Unlike the European medical marketplace, where the official role of women in medicine was restricted to pregnancy and childbirth, in central Mexico women practiced general medicine openly alongside men. Of course, they worked as midwives too—*tepalehuiani*, "the one that helps"—but the name *tícitl*, and status that went with it, applied equally to women as to men.[15] In this sense, we might imagine the Nahua midwife as an integral part of the medical establishment, not someone on the fringe of official medicine like her European counterpart; those that solicited her services for an impending birth, above all, referred to her as *tícitl*, a physician.[16] Sahagún's description of "good" and "bad" *médicas* differs little from that of male physicians: "[she knows] well the properties of herbs, and roots, trees, and stones . . . knows how to bleed, administer purges, give medicine, apply ointments, palpitate what is hard in the body to make it soft, set bones, to cup and cure sores and gout, and diseases of the eyes, and to cut small tumors from them." She, too, was skilled in interpreting and manipulating the influence that supernatural elements had on the human body: . . . "from [one's] teeth she pulls worms, and from other parts of the body, paper, flint, obsidian (*navaja de la tierra*), removing these things, she says that she cures the sick, this being a falsity and notorious superstition."[17] It is interesting to note that in cataloging the tasks of female physicians, Sahagun's informants mention various forms of eye problems, suggesting that, together with childbirth, this might have been another area of medicine overseen exclusively by women. On this same note, it is not surprising that the list for male doctors includes an item—"*dar puntos*," the stitching of wounds—that is clearly omitted in that of their female counterparts. In the warlike world of the Mexica, the *tícitl* would have been forced to be dexterous in the treatment of wounds, the repositioning of ears and noses severed on the battlefield. This type of activity and the site where it was practiced would have excluded the presence of women.[18]

Sahagún's sources have the most to say about female *titici* in their role as midwives. The Nahuas had considerable skill in the various techniques of obstetrics: they made use of numerous medications that induced and advanced labor, and produced abortions; they knew how to rotate a fetus that was not positioned correctly for a safe delivery; and they could remove a dead child (in pieces!) from the mother's womb, a last-chance effort to save her life.[19] Yet what emerges even more in the text is a sense of the enormous social importance that surrounds the birth of a child, especially a first-born, and by extension, the *tícitl*'s role as director of this process. The pregnant young woman is formally presented to the midwife's care—"she is placed in your hands, in your lap, on your back"—by her family with lavish and beautiful speech. As the physician takes charge of the pregnancy, she makes clear the "great dangers of death that lie in the interior of women" and warns the relatives to let nothing befall the expectant mother. The young woman should not "cry, or be sad, nor should anyone give her trouble," nor should she "work much, nor try to be diligent nor resourceful . . . nor run, nor tremble, nor have a fright of anything, because these things cause miscarriage." Along with these and many other earthly precautions, the *tícitl* appeals to the goddess of medicine, *Yoaltícitl* for a safe pregnancy and delivery. For the Nahuas, childbirth was something precious and sacred; the women who died giving birth to their first child were called *mochihuaquetzqui*, "valiant women," and their corpses were carried by the midwives to a grave in a special temple. So revered was this form of death that grave robbing was a problem. Soldiers believed these cadavers held unique powers; a finger from the left hand or some hair from the head brought them courage and strength when carried onto the battlefield behind their shield.[20]

In addition to the midwife, were there other medical practitioners in this Mesoamerican marketplace that specialized in particular therapies? Modern science today, at least in the West, has imposed an anatomical and pathological model of illness on the practice of medicine, so perhaps it is inappropriate to ask this question about a society that, lacking this worldview, could not possibly have had specialists in our sense of word, that is, practitioners trained in the management of diseases of one organ or system in the body.[21] Nonetheless, there does seem to be some indication that certain *titici* dedicated themselves to the treatment of specific problems, although firm evidence that would show the how and why of this is scarce. In any event, we can explore briefly a few of them here. Those curers that caused a person's illness to manifest itself in objects and then extract them through some sort of physical manipulation, usually by suction, were called *techichinani*, "those that suck." The Nahuas believed that the removal of these objects—pieces of stone, obsidian, sticks, or paper—would initiate the curing process.[22] Regaining a lost *tonalli*, a curing technique used often on sick children, was entrusted to a skilled *tetonalmacanime*. The *tonalli*—"a force that gives a person vigor, warmth, valor and allows him to grow"—was essential to good health and its absence could cause sickness, even death. *Tonalli* loss, a phenomenon that we explore in Chapter 4, could occur from any number of things: the cutting of one's hair, a sudden fright, divine punishment, or intentional harm brought about by sorcery. The *tícitl* might diagnose this condition by placing "the child over the water, and if they see the child's face dark in it, as if covered by shadow, they judge as certain" the loss of his "fate and fortune." They also used the standard divination techniques of the day, the measurement with hands or the throwing of maize kernels in water, with their tendency to float or sink carefully watched.

Remedies for *tonalli* loss included the use of incantations and medicines that "warmed" like tobacco or *tlacopatli,* a plant used to cure illnesses associated with cold.[23] Another type of *tícitl* whose services might be solicited for his or her specialized knowledge of techniques connected with the supernatural world was the *paini,* "one who drinks medicine," that is, someone skilled in the use of psychotropic drugs. More specifically, these practitioners might be grouped within the broad category of *tlaciuhgue,* those that practiced the art of fortune-telling or divination, with the intent to know events in the future, the origins of an illness, or the duration of a lifetime. The most common drugs used by the *paini* were *peyote* and *ololiuhqui,* a very powerful seed that, according to Ruiz de Alarcón, "when drunk, deprives men of judgment." The psychotropic placed its user into a trancelike state, allowing him access to realms of reality that were closed to people in ordinary states of consciousness; there, among the multiple deities that influenced daily life in Mexico, answers might be revealed not only for health problems but also for the whereabouts of lost or stolen items as well. The *paini* did not always take the powerful drug himself, but might advise the patient himself how to do so, indicating "the day and the hour in which he is to drink it, and he tells him for what purpose he will drink it." Apparently, this type of medical service did not come cheap, at least according to Ruiz de Alarcón who says of the *paini* that he "is paid very well, and they bribe him with meals and drinks in their fashion."[24]

Evidence about further specialization in the medical field is quite sketchy. Illustrations in the *Florentine Codex* show various healers associated with specific ailments: the bonesetter, *tepoztecpahtiani,* for example, the bleeder, *teitzminqui,* or the one who cures diseases of the eyes, *texpatiani.* [25] In reality, we do not know if these are examples of specialized *titici*; or, more likely, if these terms simply refer to activities that any proficient *tícitl* would have been expected to perform.

What does emerge from the sources, however, is a portrait of the Nahua physician as a person of stature and distinction in his world, a standing bestowed invariably on those who served as connection points between the gods and ordinary humans. Yet the common health care problems of everyday life also would have ensured that not all healers occupied such lofty positions, and therefore we should keep in mind the distinction between two groups of professionals: those who, trained in the temples, performed sacerdotal duties, and those who practiced the more manually oriented craft inherited from family elders. But even this latter group rated high social status. It is no accident that Sahagún, in his list of occupations, includes the physician among the artisans that the Mexica held most in high esteem (the others were the featherworker, the lapidary, and the goldsmith).[26] We also should note here that the condemnation of *médicos malos* found in these same texts, apart from the European objection to "superstitious" practices, surely include descriptions of what the Nahuas themselves considered to be "bad doctors," that is, the charlatans and the sorcerers who used their skills to inflict harm. The bad physician is "a fraud, a half-hearted worker, a killer with his medicines, a giver of overdoses, an increaser of [sickness]."[27] Likewise, the bad sorcerer is one who uses his or her considerable powers to harm and "damage the bodies [of others] with his spells, and deprives them of their judgement."[28] Unfortunately, the historical sources are silent on how those governing Nahua society dealt with these illicit practitioners. The same cannot be said, luckily, about the next phase of Mexican history, the period of Spanish rule.

HEALERS IN NEW SPAIN

Although the outlines of a medical marketplace in Mexico on the eve of the Spanish conquest are barely perceptible, they become somewhat more apparent as one moves through the three centuries of Spanish rule. Here the sources are more plentiful. Early modern Spain was a remarkably bureaucratic society for its time and its administration of its American colonies likewise generated multiple layers of government and the corresponding shuffling of papers; codes of law were promulgated through Royal decrees, Pragmatics, and Ordinances, and lawsuits abounded, leaving an abundance of historical documentation. The practice of medicine did not escape this regulatory zeal. The New World's first Protomedicato, the royal institution that regulated medical practitioners in Spain, was established in Santo Domingo in 1517. In New Spain, a royal *protomédico* was quickly appointed by the newly established town council to control the rapidly increasing numbers of practitioners already operating in the vice-regal capital.

The regulation of medical care in New Spain followed closely along lines established in the mother country. During the fifteenth and sixteenth centuries, the practice of medicine in Spain was regulated more closely than any other European country at the time.[29] Although the Protomedicato was not firmly established until the fifteenth century, Spanish medical legislation had deep roots reaching back to the Middle Ages, when many regulations designed to hold practitioners accountable were first introduced. A doctor's claim to medical knowledge he did not possess was considered a notably serious offense and fraudulent care that resulted in the patient's death could bring to the practitioner the same penalty as men who "kill treacherously" for "it is worse to poison a man than to stab him to death." The fears expressed in this legislation reflect the state of medicine at the time as much as they do the actions of healers. The wrong medicine or dosage could easily kill a patient. A surgeon might improperly use his knife or saw, or "burn his [patient's] nerves or bones so that he dies because of it." A "man or a woman" might try to make a woman pregnant with herbs but kill her instead.

Punishment for offenses such as these could be severe: a prohibition to further practice medicine, incarceration, or even death. Since the late Middle Ages, various Spanish monarchs required physicians and surgeons to demonstrate competence through examinations. Alfonso III of Aragon (1285–91) instructed the "learned and noble" to examine would-be practitioners in their "place of residence." A century later, John I of Castile (1379–90) named "*alcades mayores examinadores*" in conjunction with the "*médico primero*" of the royal household to form a body that examined such aspirants. In 1477, following Spain's unification, Ferdinand and Isabella created a central Protomedicato empowered to examine, not only physicians and surgeons but also midwives, bonesetters, apothecaries, dealers in aromatic drugs, and any other persons who "in whole or in part practice these professions"—men as well as women. The *alcades examinadores* also were given the right to try anyone for medical "crimes, excesses, and transgressions."[30]

Like other essential features of their culture, the Spanish brought their medicine with them early on in the conquest of the Americas. Just before Columbus's third voyage, Ferdinand and Isabella authorized the sending of "a physician and an apothecary and a herbalist and some instruments and sheets of music to while away the time of those people who are to be there."[31] Not long after Cortés conquered Tenochtitlan, a number of irregular healers, both locals and foreigners, began to stream into the city. Members of the newly established town council, the *cablido*, were informed of the "many persons, without being examined doctors and surgeons, [who] treat people, and because they do not know what they are doing except to relieve them of their goods, they kill some and many times leave others with many injuries and sickness . . ." Such a situation cried out for regulation. Thus, the cabildo appointed the first protomédico of New Spain in 1525 to oversee the regulation of medical practice and the precarious health of the city's inhabitants. From then on a succession of protomédicos demanded that practitioners show "by what right they practice."[32] The cabildo's right to appoint, and thus control, the protomédico might have been challenged by the crown in 1570 when the king appointed Francisco Hernández as special royal protomédico for New Spain. Philip II's instructions to the doctor consisted of two enormous tasks: first, to make a thorough survey of medicinal plants in the New World (he was supposed to move on to Peru after his time in New Spain, but, for reasons of health, he did not make it that far south), determine their curative properties, and collect samples and seeds to send back to Spain for propagation; second, as protomédico he should oversee the examination and licensing of all physcians and surgeons, and the inspection of all apothecary shops within a five-league radius of Mexico City.

Whether Hernández found his commission too onerous to apply himself fully to both sets of task or was repeatedly foiled by the town council from carrying out the latter is not entirely clear. Hernández, however, appears not to have examined a single physician or visited a single pharmacy. Instead, his seven years in Mexico were spent singularly focused on compiling his great work, the *Natural History of New Spain,* in which he describes over 3,000 native plants, birds, animals, and minerals. The cabildo, therefore, continued its oversight of the regulation and discipline of medical practitioners until 1646 when the formal machinery of the royal Protomedicato was finally set in motion.[33]

It is important to place the crown's efforts to control who practiced medicine and how in perspective. At least in theory, the power of the Protomedicato to shape the practice of medicine in New Spain was enormous. It alone was empowered to insure that the viceroyalty was cared for by qualified professionals; its charge was to eradicate the charlatans and casters of spells, the myriad curanderos, and most importantly, the countless unlicensed *empiricos* from the realm. In addition to its authority over the examination and licensing of all medical practitioners, it functioned as a tribunal, not only enforcing medical laws but adjudicating them as well. Every official action in the medical profession had to go through this body, including those pertaining to the production and sale of pharmaceuticals. Pharmacists were examined and licensed by them, and their shops, the *boticas,* were inspected on a regular basis by Protomedicato officials. But this power on paper was radically limited by conditions on the ground. Licensed physicians, surgeons, and pharmacists were woefully scarce at all times during Spanish rule. Querétaro, for example, had only two licensed doctors in 1787 to care for a population of 35,000.[34] Filling this gap was a whole spectrum of healers representing various medical traditions, from rational Galenic therapy to magically oriented medical beliefs. In Mexico City and other large towns, unlicensed practitioners flourished, and in the countryside they were dominant. As we shall see, colonial authorities themselves were mostly to blame for this shortage of legally sanctioned healers. The rigid social codes that dictated who could and could not study medicine reduced the pool of potential applicants to a handful. The structure of colonial government, too, made it difficult to get a medical license if one did not live in Mexico City, as licensing could take place only in the capital. Throughout the whole period of Spanish rule, then, the panorama of medical specialists consisted of a small number of university trained practitioners competing with a multitude of popular European and native healers. For convenience sake, this exploration of the medical marketplace examines these healers separately, but the artificiality of this will soon become apparent; the lines between the different sorts of practitioners was quite blurred, even among the licensed professionals.

LICENSED PRACTITIONERS

PHYSICIANS

For well-off city dwellers—the wealthy Spanish and creole families—there was an integrated pyramid of practitioners to choose from. At the top was the *médico* or university educated physician. In theory, médicos were concerned only with "internal medicine" such as fevers and epidemic diseases, whereas "external medicine," the treatment of wounds, broken limbs, and amputations, fell to the surgeon. Medicine in the sixteenth century was an integral part of science and philosophy, therefore its practitioners were part of the intellectual elite that disdained any association with a "mechanical" craft.[35] Medical education in New Spain, as in the mother country, stressed a rational orientation to matters of health and illness that appealed primarily to *gente de razón*, the "rational people" of the upper and middle classes. For the vast majority of New Spain's population—indigenous peoples, blacks, mestizos, mulattos, and poor whites—being sick continued to have a supernatural significance that no reference to the rational workings of the humors could fully explain. "For these people, eloquence and debating skills, philosophical argumentation and flawless quotations of texts sharpened through numerous examinations and *oposiciones*, meant little. Hippocrates had indeed come to the colonies, but he was known only among the educated elite."[36]

Shortage of legal medical care was endemic throughout Spain's three-hundred-year-rule in the Americas. Colonial sources show that in 1545 there were apparently only four certified doctors in the entire capital of New Spain. One of them, Cristóbal Méndez, had recently been arrested by the Inquisition on charges of sorcery; another, Juan de Alcázar, was preparing to return to Castile. That left only the licentiate Pedro López and Pedro de la Torre, a man who had recently fled Vera Cruz on charges of practicing without a license.[37] Over two hundred years later, every city and town of importance in New Spain still suffered a shortage of licensed physicians. Between 1607 and 1738, the University of Mexico granted 438 bachelors' degrees in medicine, an average of 3.35 a year.[38] Such numbers fell well below the needs of the country.

Why the chronic shortage of licensed physicians in New Spain? Like their counterparts in Spain, the colonial authorities greatly limited the pool of health care professionals eligible for certification by the Protomedicato. All prospective physicians and surgeons were subject to strict laws regarding their legitimacy and blood purity or *limpieza de sangre*. Such laws originated from Spain's recent and not-so-recent past. In late medieval Spain a large number of Jews and Moors were prominent physicians; they occupied important posts at the royal court, took care of clergymen, and worked as municipal physicians. After the Catholic Kings expelled the Jews in 1492, *limpieza de sangre* became a requirement for anyone desiring to practice medicine. Shortly thereafter, Moors and Moriscos were restricted from entering universities and thus prohibited from legally practicing medicine. It was this climate of racial and religious intolerance, especially during the late-sixteenth-century Counter-Reformation, that aggravated the already acute shortage of legal health care workers in Spain.[39] The meaning of *limpieza de sangre* took on new implications in the Indies. Statues of the University of Mexico stated early on that no blacks, mulattos, *chino morenos*, or any kind of slave or former slaves were to be permitted to enter the university. Native Mexicans were equally unacceptable.[40] In addition, the geographical centralization of the Protomedicato in Mexico City—no regional offices or examine sites were ever set up during the colonial period—meant that even those lawfully trained in some form of the medical arts would have to make the long and costly journey to the capital in order to receive a license.

Given the critical need for qualified medical practitioners, it is surprising how long it took before medical education was established in New Spain. The *primera* chair of medicine, named in accordance with conical hours, was first created in 1578, almost three decades after the founding of the University of Mexico. Twenty years later, a second chair of medicine, *visperas*, followed. Students received two one-hour lectures per day in which professors dictated in Latin from a classical text in front of them; for the rest of the hour the lecturer explained the text, occasionally in the vernacular. This was a highly formalized curriculum that was purely theoretical. For four years, students read the works of Hippocrates, Galen, and Avicenna on humoral theory, temperaments, the nature of man, fevers, and pulse. In 1621, responding to a decree issued by Philip III, who wanted to improve medical education both at home and in the colonies, the University of Mexico founded two more chairs. One, *Metodo Medendi*, or therapeutic methodology, was based on Galen's text of the same name; the other chair was *Anatomía*, offering instruction in anatomy and surgery. Only then did the first university in the Americas fully qualify under Spanish law to train and graduate bachelors, licenciates, and doctors of medicine.

The legal requirements and process of acquiring the medical degree remained fairly stable from the sixteenth to the nineteenth century. By the time a man—women not having yet the legal right to higher education—had obtained the bachelor's degree of medicine, the *Bachiller de Medicina,* he had already spent eight years in the university, four earning the bachelor's degree and four studying medicine. After an additional two years of internship with an established physician, the candidate might present himself to the royal Protomedicato for examination. Because the bachelor of arts degree consumed the years that, in current American terms, would be the period devoted to high school, the Mexican student would be ready to enter medical school at about the age the modern student enters college. Thus, he could finish his professional training at the time the modern student graduates from college—in his mid-twenties—and be fully qualified to practice medicine. Two other degrees in medicine were possible, the licentiate and the doctorate. Only the *licenciatura* required further study, mostly the reading and committing to memory of more classic texts required to perform the "acts" and stand the long and grueling examinations. The doctoral degree required no further studies, only an additional exam, and in some cases was conferred on the candidate only a few days after the licentiate. The main difference between the two seemed to be one of status rather than knowledge; such status was clearly on display in the very expensive and elaborate ceremony in which the doctoral candidate participated in as part of his graduation.[41]

SURGEONS

Although more humble in status than the physician, the surgeon played a more ample role in New Spain's medical marketplace. Surgery was considered a manual craft rather than an intellectual science, involving the hand, not the head. The *cirujano* treated external ailments such as wounds and injuries, broken bones, and skin conditions such as boils and rashes. He also typically pulled teeth, let blood, and treated kidney stones, hernias, and venereal diseases. Surgeons constituted a very broad spectrum of practitioners in New Spain. The surgeon's world was easier to enter than the physician's; but once inside, many cirujanos easily passed over into the practice of "internal" medicine, which was more prestigious and lucrative. Much of everyday practice was in the hands of barber surgeons, *cirujanos barberos,* who considerably outnumbered physicians and had an important role in what today would be considered primary medical care. Surely it was surgeons, not physicians, that came in the first ships to the Indies, and later accompanied the conquistadores. Bernal Díaz mentions one of them, a "Maestre Juan," who is called by Pánfilo Narváez after a battle to tend to his wounded eye. Later on, after the fall of Tenochtitlan, the same surgeon is still on the scene, curing the wounded at "excessive prices."[42]

Colonial officials employed surgeons early on to treat the incarcerated and the poor. In 1525 the newly formed *Ayuntamiento* in Mexico approved the amount of 50 pesos annually for Francisco Soto, "barber and surgeon, so that he should reside in this city and perform those services."[43] And in 1610, just three years after it began appointing physicians to treat the poor, the cabildo of Mexico City began to hire barber surgeons as well.[44] The Inquisition continually employed medical personal—physicians, barber surgeons, nurses, and midwives—to attend the prisoners in its jails. The vast records of the Mexican Holy Office often note when a doctor or surgeon had attended a certain prisoner, but in a few cases more detail was given. One such case is that of Teresa Romero, a young woman accused of being an *alumbrada*, someone who claims to be in direct communication with God. Although she was only 18 years old and unmarried ("*se hallaba en opinión de doncella*") at the time she entered the Inquisition's prison, she was eight months pregnant. A midwife was brought in to oversee the delivery, along with an Indian woman who had recently given birth to attend the new mother and child. For the next ten years, Teresa (along with her son!) lived in a dark cell while awaiting her trial, and on many occasions she requested medical care for herself and the child. On one occasion she complained of "*vómitos de cólera*," for which the *médico*, a Doctor de los Arcos, prescribed a concoction made from peach pits, and for her son, who was suffering from a rash, an ointment of animal fat. And, at various times, a surgeon was called in to perform bleedings on Teresa.[45]

Another document from the Inquisition provides insight into the kinds of medical services surgeons actually provided. In the 1640s, Juan de Correa, "*Barbero y Cirujano de las Cárceles Secretas del Santo Oficio*," petitioned the tribunal for more pay by enumerating the services he had provided. In five years of service, he claimed to have performed over 4,000 shaves, at least 1,200 bleedings, pulled 37 teeth, applied 90 pairs of cupping glasses (*ventosas*), opened and cured 32 ulcers, and succored the "tortured" and "whipped" (*atormentados y azotados*). In addition to these typical surgeons' tasks, he also claimed to have treated successfully hundreds of ailments and illnesses (*achaques y enfermedades*), all with the "utmost care, certainty, and study."[46] In theory, the line separating médicos from cirujanos was clearly marked, in everyday practice it was not.

The wide gulf separating the elite physician and humble surgeon was common to most parts of Europe. Although physicians of the ancient world were expected to be competent in both medicine and surgery, from the late Middle Ages until the eighteenth century the two were the province of separate groups of practitioners. Universities controlled the licensing of physicians, while surgeons were regulated by the trade guilds. Because the surgeon's closest occupational links were with the barbers, it became common for the two trades to be carried on by a single practitioner, the barber-surgeon. The earliest guilds of barber-surgeons date back to the thirteenth century. In 1540, the Surgeons of

London united with the Barber-Surgeons' Company becoming one of the largest guilds in the city. Guild members had strong economic incentives to control the numbers of would-be practitioners entering the trade and ensure a basic level of competence by apprenticeship. Spanish barber-surgeons differed from their northern European counterparts in that they, ostensibly at least, operated under the control of the centralized Protomedicato, and thus were not organized into trade guilds that set their profession apart from other medical practitioners. In fact, one recent study argues persuasively that reforms under Philip II created a more positive environment of exchange—of knowledge and techniques—between university educated practitioners and empirically trained barber-surgeons than existed in other countries of Europe at the time.[47]

Although it appears that most European surgeons were of the mechanical arts variety—trained by apprenticeship to treat the accidents and injuries of daily life—a few came out of a separate tradition of academic surgery that had flourished in southern Europe since the late Middle Ages. This was especially true in the universities of Italy where surgical theory and anatomy were taught by physicians. Because of the links between the Crown of Aragon and the leading Italian universities, this tradition of surgical scholarship gradually spread into Spain. During the sixteenth century medical faculty at Spanish institutions, such as the universities of Alcalá de Henares and Valencia, enthusiastically adopted the teachings of Andreas Versalius (1514–64), the great anatomist, along with the practice of human dissections that would eventually enrich theoretical knowledge of disease. A new generation of academic surgeons emerged at this time and made significant contributions to contemporary surgical literature. It was this development, combined with the reforms of Philip II making surgical study part of the medical curriculum, that allowed surgery to achieve a social and professional status in Renaissance Spain perhaps unequaled in Europe at that time.[48] But the flowering of Spanish surgery was brief. Toward the end of the sixteenth century, innovative scholarship in medicine and surgery declined for reasons that are still being explored by historians today. Explanations of Spain's perceived "backwardness" in science and technology—the origins of which are often traced to the late fifteenth and sixteenth centuries—are plentiful: the censorship of a powerful and exceptionally active church; a culture shaped by a long history of religious crusading that valued warriors and clergy above other callings; the statues of purity of blood to exclude persons of Jewish or Muslim ancestry from entering universities; Philip II's 1558 prohibition of Spanish students studying outside the Spanish kingdoms; and, perhaps most important, the overextension of Spanish resources as Philip fought several costly wars—in Tripoli, Malta, the Low Countries, the disastrous Armada loss—which severely limited Spain's ability to play a part in the seventeenth-century scientific revolution.[49]

Ideas about the education of surgeons began to change in the eighteenth century signaling the beginning of the end of surgical training by apprenticeship. The surgical elite in Europe, and later in Spanish America, sought to raise professional standards in accordance with the various ideological and economic changes taking place during the Enlightenment. The emphasis on observation and experimentation increased the respectability of the methods of the surgeon, which now came to be frequently combined with academic theories of medicine. University courses and medical degrees gradually supplanted apprenticeship and guild certification, making surgery, obstetrics, and ophthalmology medical specialties rather than lower-status occupations. Much of this new education was carried out in conjunction with the hospital and the state. The latter, often through the military and/or private interests, established (or transformed) hospitals into exclusively medical institutions (rather than the shelters of Christian charity they had been since the Middle Ages) to treat the chronically or acutely ill, the injured, and, increasingly common in the latter part of the century, to deliver babies, and to train medical practitioners, primarily surgeons. Hospital training ideally combined the surgical apprentice's hands-on experience with the medical pupil's theoretical analysis of individual cases.[50] In Spain, the first Royal College of Surgery was established in Cádiz in 1748. Shortly thereafter, other surgical colleges were established in Barcelona and Madrid. Because the Bourbon monarchy at this time made the modernization of the military a priority, the new surgical schools were designed to cater to the needs of the growing army and navy. In addition, the power of the Spanish state was enhanced by breaking the monopoly of the universities and limiting the power of the Royal Protomedicato. In eighteenth-century Mexico, as in Spain, a fresh interest in surgery and anatomy was on the rise. The Real Escuela de Cirugía was established in 1768, modeled on the new surgical institutions in the Peninsula. Its founding was part of the Bourbon state's reorganization of its colonies, and the school was very closely linked to the needs of the military in New Spain.[51]

In Spain, and by extension its American colonies, surgeons were usually distinguished by educational background: the *cirujano latino*, the long-gowned surgeon, university trained and well versed in Latin, and the *cirujano romancista*, the short-gowned surgeon, lacking both a knowledge of Latin and a formal education. This distinction was carried over into the regulations governing medical practice in New Spain, although much uncertainty has surrounded the question of qualifications to practice as a romance surgeon. During the colonial period, most surgeons practicing with a license had at least four or five years of apprenticeship in a hospital or, lacking that, under the tutelage of some "approved" surgeon who, most likely, acquired his skills in the same way. Like the candidate for physician, the aspiring surgeon also had to produce the necessary documents establishing *limpieza de sangre*, a certificate of baptism, and documents of good character and habits. After the establishment of the Real Escuela de Cirugía in the eighteenth century, no student was allowed to be associated with a barbershop, which "would lead him into vicious habits out of keeping with the honor and respect due to the faculty he was entering." And even though most candidates did not enter the school with a bachelor's degree in medicine—thus, they could not be considered Latin surgeons—their graduation from such an institution stipulated that they were not romance surgeons either.[52]

Although surgeons were disdained by physicians, they surface frequently in the records, suggesting that they were much more commonly consulted than their elite competitors. These were the general practitioners of their day. The more one reads the contemporary documents, the more evident it becomes that the category of medical practitioners called surgeons is a very large and fluid one. Various levels of official medicine were practiced by people calling themselves *cirujanos*, many of them specializing in the treatment of specific problems that demanded practical skills: the *algebrista*, or bone-setter, who set fractures and reduced dislocations; the *sacador de la piedra*, who removed painful bladder stones; the *hernista*, who reduced and managed hernias; and the *batidor de la catarata*, or oculist, who specialized in treating cataracts.[53] Both bone setters and oculists were appointed at various times in the sixteenth and seventeenth centuries by the cabildo in Mexico City to treat the poor.[54]

At the lower echelons of surgery were the phlebotomists or bleeders, popularly called *barberos*. The use of bloodletting was a major feature of Greek rational medicine, and although surgeons, and some physicians, performed this technique, barbers were the "technicians" who specialized in the procedure known as *sangrías*. Although required by law to be licensed, bleeders were not expected to have academic training or even to be literate but only to have apprenticed with an approved surgeon or phlebotomist for four years. What *barberos* actually did may be deduced from the kind of questions the protomédicos asked the phlebotomist seeking a license. A solid knowledge of veins and arteries was crucial in order to bleed properly and to apply the cupping glasses and leeches. But exam questions indicate that barberos were not limited to bloodletting alone. It seems he was also expected to know how to lance boils and treat ulcers, how to handle accident victims, and how to extract teeth, especially troublesome molars—a handy skill in an age before modern dentistry significantly reduced tooth decay.[55]

Like other branches of the colonial medical profession, phlebotomists were a diverse group. The upper crust of practitioners were licensed and many of them owned their own shop, or *tienda*, or managed one for a colleague. Slightly beneath them were those barbers that, although not licensed by the Protomedicato, had been legitimately apprenticed in their craft; many of these, too, owned or worked in shops. More numerous, however, were the lower orders of the trade: the unlicensed bleeders who did not work at established tiendas but offered their services in *puestos* at the various open markets that dotted the urban landscape of New Spain. In a very early description of colonial Mexico City, Francisco Cervantes de Salazar mentions that the barbers operated out of stalls with "all classes of artisans and craftsmen"—carpenters, locksmiths, shoemakers, weavers, and breadmakers—along the *calle de Tacuba*.[56] Another chronicler from the eighteenth century mentions that the barber stands were among those removed from the *Plaza de Volador* anytime there were bullfights; the barbers there, it was noted by another, "set themselves up [and] apply their skill to the poor who come to be bled or to have their beard cut."[57] Bleeders also set up shop "beyond the walls" of the city to escape detection by the authorities. Run by so-called *chinos*, these shops so greatly increased in number that in 1636 the viceroy, the Marquis of Cadereyta, gave strict orders that no more than twelve of these should be allowed to operate. As with most laws clamping down on the illegal practice of medicine, this appears to have had little effect; fourteen years later, a similar order was issued again by another viceroy.[58]

The barbershop must have been a common sight in colonial Mexico City. According to a survey of phlebotomists in 1790, there were a total of eighty-six registered tiendas operating in the capital.[59] Numerous other small shops must have existed in the recesses of the city, beyond the reach of authorities. Although *barberos* were thick on the ground, it is not clear whether they all practiced the medical craft of bleeding, cupping, applying leeches, and pulling teeth. But because those who did were supposed to be licensed, the Protomedicato stipulated that *sangradores* should distinguish themselves from those barbers that only trimmed and shaved beards. Over the centuries, in both Spain and its American colonies, *ordenanzas* were issued so that "pure Barbers not be confused with bleeders, and [so that] the Public does not suffer from errors on this point, . . . the former should indispensably display in the doors of their shops a curtain and basin, [and] the latter should distinguish their shops as always with a lattice window and tile (*celosía y tejar*), [it] being understood that the Barbers, if they exceed [their position] by bleeding or pulling teeth, the Visitador del Protomedicato will proceed against them in accordance with the laws." At one point, there was also an attempt made to have those barbers who worked in the city streets ("*en aire libre*") to wear a large hat with a white feather in order to be identified as medical attendants. This suggestion met with little success and bleeders continued, for the most part, without regulation.[60]

A surviving inventory from 1575 gives us the opportunity to imagine the inside of a barber's tienda and to know something about the barber himself. The shop, located on Tacuba Street, belonged to the barber-surgeon Alonso Salas, who was arrested by the Inquisition for insulting an official of that body (*injurias a la Autoridad*). The tienda must have been a decent-sized operation, as it had three barber's chairs, all made from orange-wood, a large mirror, at least twelve brass and silver basins, several decorative wall hangings (*guadamaciles de cuero colorado*), leather-covered boxes filled with small surgical and shaving tools, plus a large assortment of razors, knives, and lancets. We can surmise from the inventory too that Salas was probably a literate man as his goods included four books on surgery, a book of stories, and two hand-painted writing desks. We also know that he was a man of higher status in this colonial world because he traveled about on horseback. In addition to the personal goods of his household, Salas owned a bay horse and a dark pony with saddle and bridle plus other riding tack such as iron stirrups, spurs, and a breast plate decorated with bells. This barber was well-armed, too, owning several guns (*una escopeta y un arcabus*) and a sword. Obviously Salas moved in circles of higher standing in Mexico City, at least until his arrest by the Inquisition.[61]

PHARMACISTS

Parallel in status to the surgeon was the *boticario*, or pharmacist. Ostensibly limited by the Protomedicato to preparing and selling the simples and compounds that were the staples of colonial medicine, in reality many boticarios practiced some kind of medicine. Boticarios occupied a unique position in New Spain's medical marketplace. For one, unlike many of the surgeons that practiced in colonial Mexico, pharmacists were usually literate and had some knowledge of Latin. This gave them access not only to information on preparing medicines from various botanical and animal materials but also to books written on the diagnosis and treatment of diseases. In addition, their specialized training—like that of surgeons, a four-year apprenticeship—gave them access to imported and local medicines, and, at least by law, the exclusive right to sell them to the public as the pharmacy, or *botica*, was the only establishment that was licensed to sell the public ready-made medicines or have a physician's prescription filled. In addition to literacy in Latin, the pharmacist needed to demonstrate a solid knowledge of the medicinal properties of several hundred plants, along with numerous animals and minerals. To transformation these ingredients into medicines for public consumption the he would need to master the different methods of preparing the simples and compounds, such as infusion, sublimation, filtration, and distillation. In addition to his pharmacological skills, the boticario seeking a license had to prove, of course, his *limpieza de sangre* with documents that showed that none of his ancestors were of Jewish, Moorish, Indian, or African blood.[62]

Among the many laws that governed boticas in the cities of New Spain, were a number of restrictions on who could own them. Both physicians and surgeons were prohibited from owning boticas just as pharmacists were not legally allowed to practice medicine. One way that the Protomedicato sought to keep abuses in the practice of medicine low was to separate the functions of practitioners. Thus, surgeons and physicians should not have a financial interest in the treatments they prescribe, nor should pharmacists be able to profit from the sale of drugs they themselves recommended. In addition, a boticario was not allowed to own more than one pharmacy, even if it were in a different town.[63]

A further restriction on ownership was one that made it illegal for women to own pharmacies. As in other areas of the practice of medicine, these laws governing the dispensing of drugs did not reflect everyday reality. For one thing, some women did own boticas, even though the law forbade them to operated "either publicly or secretly," even with a licensed boticario filling prescriptions, a prohibition that remained on the books until 1801, when women were allowed to own, but not manage, pharmacies.[64] A late-eighteenth-century survey shows that at least five out of the thirty-five pharmacies surveyed in Mexico City belonged to women.[65] Other cases surface in the colonial sources of women fighting in the courts to retain the right to operate the shops they had inherited from deceased fathers or husbands. One such instance occurred in Celaya during the waning years of Spanish rule. The botica that Doña Ana de Aponte had inherited from her parents, and had been in her family for more than twenty years, was closed by local authorities "with no other idea than the welfare of the public" in mind, and on the allegation that the *boticario* in charge did not have a proper license. For the next three years, from 1801 to 1804, Doña Ana went through the long, drawn-out process of appealing her case, first to the district court of Querétaro, and finally to the Protomedicato itself in Mexico City. The source of her undoing, most likely, was her only competition in town: a botica owned by a surgeon, also in clear violation of the law. Doña Ana claimed that the local, and later, the regional officials and inspectors were in collusion with the surgeon and biased against her. The records are silent on whether or not her persistence was rewarded.[66] And despite the law prohibiting her competitor from owning a pharmacy, this appears to have been a fairly common phenomenon for both surgeons and physicians. The bachiller Jan Manuel Venegas and Pedro Puglia, both brought before the authorities on charges of dispensing drugs illegally, were a few of the many physicians who owned pharmacies in the late eighteenth century.[67]

Probably the most frequent violators of the Protomedicato's pharmaceutical laws were the pharmacists themselves. Although strictly prohibited from practicing medicine, most boticarios not only gave medical advice, but treated their clients' illnesses as well. So commonplace was this practice that a pharmacist did not hesitate to sue a client for nonpayment of fees. In 1779, the boticario, Manuel del Castillo, filed suit against one of his former patients, Bartolomé de Martos, for not paying his medical bills. The case, which was brought before the authorities of the Criminal Court of the Province of Mexico, goes into a fair amount of detail about the illnesses of Don Bartolome, his wife, and two daughters, all treated at their home by the boticario over a period of one year and seven months. These ailments—Don Bartolome's diarrhea and *insultos*, a temporary attack of paralysis; Doña Maria Micaela de Sierra's paralysis in her legs, and the daughters, Maria Luisa and Maria Micaela, both nuns in local convents, painful kidney stones—were conditions that, ostensibly at least, would have fallen under the purview of the surgeon and the physician. But the pharmacist was well placed to compete with his high-status competitors; he had unequaled access to foreign and local medicines and the knowledge to prepare them, and, because he was literate, access to medical books that would direct him in diagnosis and treatment. This combination assured him an important place in the medical marketplace.[68]

In addition to overseeing examinations and licensing, the Protomedicato was charged with carrying out periodic inspections, or *visitias*, of all the pharmacies in its jurisdiction, that is, all those public boticas, whether privately owned or part of a hospital or religious institution, in relatively urban areas. The *visita* was supposed to ensure that pharmacists were operating with a proper license, that medicines were being prepared and dispensed correctly, that the shop was properly stocked with the basic ingredients, that the boticario was not overcharging the public, and, most important, to ensure that medicines were not "corrupted or altered." The pharmacopeia commonly used in New Spain, apart from the addition of several native medicines, was not that much different from that being used in Europe. The large number of remedies available, from simple herbs to the most complex preparations, were divided into *simples* and *compuestas*. The former included any single organic material—animal, plant, or mineral—used alone as medicine or employed in the preparation of a compound. The compuestas were medicines prepared from a variety of simples. Since medicines were derived almost completely from plants or animal materials they were prone to spoilage rather quickly. The offense of selling medicine past its prime or, worst yet, selling one that had been altered and sold under false pretense was considered especially serious by Protomedicato authorities and the general public alike. Such medicines were confiscated and burned publicly, and the boticario was order to replace them with "medicines of good quality," and fined 6,000 maravedís.[69]

This description conforms pretty much with the experience of one seventeenth-century boticario named Blas de Naveda. A routine *visita* by two members of the Protomedicato, a scribe, and a local pharmacist, to his tienda quickly uncovered the fact that it lacked many of the basic staples of pharmacology. When asked to produce his oils, Naveda could show nothing but a little rose-colored oil. Of the essential purges and "usuals," he could only show endive, borage, and roses. When asked to display common ointments made from gourds, lead, sandalwood, and tutty, he could not do so. In addition to the serious deficit of supplies, there were reports of Naveda's bad "preservation" and preparation of his drugs. Apparently, this was not the first time that authorities had found serious problems in Naveda's shop, yet despite repeated inspections and warnings he had not made the slightest improvements. This last inspection sealed the case against Naveda; his botica was closed and he was promptly thrown into jail to await trial. Ten days after the inspection, his "damaged" medicines burned in the "Plaza Mayor of this city next to the gallows," and his license suspended for four years, Blas de Naveda was formally released from jail.[70]

MIDWIVES

At the very fringe of official medicine was the midwife. Although they operated without being licensed, I include them here because, ostensibly at least, the Protomedicato had jurisdiction over them; their practice was not illegal (unless they were found using "superstitious" methods), but no real effort was made to regulate them either. Two facts concerning the *partera* or *matrona* are remarkable when considered together: practically every child in Mexico, at least well into the nineteenth century, was delivered by a midwife, and yet we know almost nothing about them. The need for their services was so widespread and common—fertility rates for women in Colonial Mexico have been estimated at about 8.5 births[71]—that it was rarely mentioned.

Two reasons account for this indifference: the birth of a child was not yet viewed as a medical event, and pregnancy and childbirth took place in a world confined exclusively to women. Throughout most of the colonial period, the *partera* or *matrona* was free to practice and her role in assisting women with childbirth was rarely questioned by the Protomedicato. Only in cases of difficult deliveries, which most often resulted in the death of the mother, child, or both, was the colonial midwife bound by any sort of legislation; in such a case it obliged her to seek a surgeon's aid for the suffering parturient. Parteras, too, sometimes were subject to Inquisitional scrutiny for practices that had any appearance of witchcraft or idolatry. In 1617, Doña Ana de Angulo was brought before the tribunal for giving a woman in labor *peyote* and placing scissors under her pillow to avert afterpains. In late-eighteenth-century Pachuca, midwives came to the attention of the Inquisition for inscribing certain verses on wafers which were then feed to women in childbed, a practice "very common to this place."[72] The art and technique of midwifery in Mexico was passed down through the female line from one generation to the next, blending indigenous and European practices and beliefs. By the end of the colonial period both traditions had combined into a unique synthesis that, for the majority of Mexican women, remained the most common form of managing childbirth well into the twentieth century.

Throughout much of human history the two most significant events in the life cycle, birth and death—today both highly medicalized—were not seen as medical events, and their management was very much in the hands of lay and religious experts. Studies of childbirth in early modern England, where more testimony about their practices have survived, have shown that it was a highly ritualized social ceremony that was confined exclusively to women, men being rigorously excluded. Well before she went into labor, the expectant mother had already made arrangements for the birth by choosing the birth attendants—her midwife and a carefully selected group of other women , the "gossips," who would help manage the delivery. The birth included a number of rituals, dutifully carried out by the gossips, which gave ceremonial importance to the event such as the preparation of the lying-in chamber, transformed from its everyday appearance by physically and symbolically enclosing it; the preparation of the *caudle*, a hot, sweet drink made of wine or gruel and flavored with spices, which the mother drank to keep up her strength and spirits; and, after a successful delivery, the proper swaddling of the infant and the handing it over to the mother. Each midwife had her own style of managing the birth: some used force and manipulation, whereas others left things to nature; some used magic and charms, others did not; many specialized in different body postures that would help facilitate birth.[73] Midwives did not offend female modesty—a continual concern being the indecency of having men attend women in childbirth—and some of them developed considerable skills in dealing with complications. European obstetrical customs were very reminiscent of those practiced in precontact Mexico.

Midwives in New Spain officiated over the birth very much like their European counterparts. These were almost always older women, usually widowed.[74] They were assisted by a couple of female attendants, called *tenedoras*, who helped position and manipulate the woman in labor. The most common positions in which Mexican women, of all backgrounds, delivered their babies were either kneeling or sitting on the birthing chair. The latter, *la silla para el parto*, which was a piece of equipment that belonged to the *partera*, was essentially a chair without a complete bottom through which the child was delivered. A variant of the kneeling position, "found among the Indians and lower classes around San Luis Postosí," had the laboring woman partially suspend herself from a rope attached to a diagonally placed beam. The midwife, situated in front of the parturient, would massage the uterus, while the *tenedora* supported her from the back. Other rituals of childbirth depended on the social groups of the participants. Mestizo and creole women, for example, might keep images of virgins or saints close to their bodies while in labor; San Ramón was a favorite among expectant mothers. During the most dangerous time of the delivery—when the child is passing through the birth canal—pieces of ribbon, paper, or religious wafers containing "words of the Virgin" might be laid on her belly.[75]

As the regulation of medicine by the state increased, the independence and autonomous practice of female midwives was curtailed. This process began in Europe in the late eighteenth century. Knowledge of obstetrics made substantial advances during this period; by the end of the century the anatomy of the gravid uterus and the physiological mechanism of normal labor, along with its three stages, had been described. The normal process of placental separation was also explained, changing ideas on the management of the dangerous third stage of labor. The older method of *accouchement forcée*, the forcible dilation of the cervix in order to speed up labor, was now condemned. Almost none of this had been known in 1700. By 1750 there were substantial numbers of "men-midwives" delivering babies in England and by the end of the century, most surgeon-apothecaries, and well as some physicians and surgeons were doing the same.[76] In Mexico these kinds of changes in how babies were delivered came much later; only in the last half of the nineteenth century did it become more common for doctors and surgeons to be involved in childbirth, and even then mostly for upper- and middle-class women. There is very little in the historical record to show that colonial authorities made any real attempt to formally educated and license midwives in New Spain, even though complaints about them were common, especially in the last half of the eighteenth century. In 1793, for example, professors at the University of Mexico repeatedly stated the need for regulation of midwifery; the surgeon and "master of anatomy," Miguel Moreno y Peña testified to the cabildo in Mexico City that "the swollen crowd of women who have introduced themselves into this city" practice at the expense of the lives of mothers and fetuses. But chronic financial stringency and an apparent lack of interest in the exclusively female world of childbirth prevented any effective response to the need for reform until well into the nineteenth century.[77]

UNLICENSED PRACTITIONERS

For the greater part of New Spain's inhabitants, regular access to medical practitioners outside of the family would have been limited to the lower echelons of official medicine—that is, to the barber surgeon, the poorer boticario, and the midwife—or to someone who fell clearly within the illegal practice of medicine such as the curandero. For the purposes of this study, I have made a distinction between legal and illegal practitioners, but such a distinction would not have mattered much to most of colonial Mexico's population. Unlicensed practitioners—sometimes called *intrusos*, or "intruders" by the authorities, were not a marginal group; rather, they formed a large and heterogeneous majority whose services were in high demand by the public. In contrast, the medical establishment was a small minority attempting to exert control over its profession. This was difficult for reasons already alluded to earlier in this chapter. Spanish authorities attempted to establish a medical system that was developed according to metropolitan models, a system that was severely challenged by the vast territories and large populations of the New World. The severe shortage of licensed medical professionals that prevailed throughout the entire colonial period quite predictably created a large vacuum into which unlicensed, and often untrained, individuals swarmed. Furthermore, the primitive state of medicine made it more difficult for the medical establishment to offer unique and superior services. The years spanning Spanish rule in Mexico took place in an environment where lay-oriented information—as opposed to the expert-oriented information of our own time—still prevailed, and medicine had not yet become the esoteric body of knowledge that would later make it the monopoly of highly trained specialists. The novice could acquire all sorts of medical expertise empirically by working alongside the barber-surgeon, the partera, and the curandero. And for the literate layman who had access to medical books and some training, the opportunities to offer services comparable to the university trained physician or surgeon—in effect to pass themselves off as licensed professionals—were abundant.

The protomédicos complained frequently that their enforcement outside of the capital was being undermined by local authorities who protected illegal practitioners. Yet, given the persistent scarcity of licensed medical professionals, municipal and regional officials were faced with two alternatives: allow large segments of the population to go without any health care at all, or, interpret the law prudently by tolerating some unlicensed healers to operate. One essential question in this larger debate was whether Indian towns fell under the same laws as those with sizable Spanish and Hispanized populations. According to the *Recopilación de Leyes*, the massive compilation of laws governing Spain's possessions in the Indies, the Protomedicato's rule on the licensing of medical practitioners only applied to "places where Spanish people live, not for Indian places."[78] When Philip IV was informed in 1652 that illegal practitioners far outnumbered their legal counterparts, his orders to Viceroy Enríquez de Guzmán made a clear distinction between unlicensed practice in Indian towns and those in which Spaniards lived. *Intrusos* in Spanish towns should be vigorously prosecuted, although, he noted in the same *real cédula*, it was not illegal to practice medicine in Indian towns without a license.[79] In an eighteenth-century lawsuit, in which the issue of healers in Indian towns was challenged, the Justice of the Indian village of Teocoaltiche in the Audencia of Guadalajara, argued that the licensing requirement should not be applied to curanderos in Indian communities because even though they did at times "act as doctors or surgeons," it was better to have "someone who has modest experience or knowledge to attend to such things, than to have an absolute lack of recourse [for help] and to be required to put oneself in the hands of people who have no understanding and lack entirely any practical knowledge."[80]

These same arguments were made time and again regarding towns with a strong Spanish and mestizo presence, especially in those sparsely populated areas in north central Mexico. Regional cabildos, faced with the paucity of legal practitioners, either licensed those with dubious qualifications, or neglected to demand their papers. In 1795, for example, a surgeon named José Sánchez Camaño, who had been practicing for two months in the Valle de Santiago, located in the intendancy of Guanajuato, protested that a horde of curanderos, bleeders, and old women were allowed to practice freely. Local authorities defended their tacit tolerance of the situation by admitting there may have been "some misfortunes," but in places where there were no examined physicians, people had to rely on those who had empirical knowledge or reading ability, and thus could prescribe or apply some simple remedies for common ailments. The outcome of this case is even more illuminating: when the Protomedicato checked the accuser's background, they found that he himself was unlicensed! The affair ended with the arrest of Sánchez Camaño and not in the ruin of the local *intrusos*.[81]

The difficulties in restraining the activities of unlicensed practitioners are further illustrated by the case of Nicolás García Miranda, a surgeon who practiced both surgery and medicine in the late eighteenth century. First exposed to medicine while working at the botica of an uncle, García Miranda later enrolled and completed four years of training at the Escuela de Cirugía, although he never obtained a license from the Protomedicato. And even though the law forbade his working in the pharmacy, he continued to do so, offering medical advice and building up a good-sized roster of patients through word of mouth. In 1784, García Miranda was fined 50 pesos and forced to leave his uncle's botica. Eight years later, the Protomedicato caught up with him again, this time for "curing people without a license." It also was noted that he treated "medical diseases" and prescribed internal medicines, areas of medicine that fell clearly outside his expertise as a surgeon. His case is interesting, more for the light it sheds on the public's perception of what constituted a qualified practitioner, than for what it says about the Protomedicato's doomed efforts at controlling the practice of medicine. Some of García Miranda's patients who testified in the case stated that he was more skillful than many licensed practitioners. One man, a José Medina, testified that he was successfully treated by the surgeon for a broken leg, whereas his wife, María Juana Estolinque, was cured of "gangrene" in her hand and legs. She had been "mutilated" and written off as a terminal case by several licensed practitioners before García Miranda took charge of her care. Another witness in the case declared that his wife, who had been gravely ill with dysentery and eventually died from her affliction, had been treated by García Miranda and a licensed physician. Despite the death of his wife, this witness felt that both practitioners had given excellent and comparable treatment, as his willingness to testify on behalf of García Miranda makes clear.[82]

Another type of intruder that inspired royal officials to mandate more laws regulating medicine was the foreign practitioner, both the legitimately trained and the fraud. The foreign doctor's prospects in New Spain were enhanced not only by the paucity of formally trained practitioners offering services, but by his European allure as well. This was as true in Spain as in its colonies. Benito Gerónimo Feijóo, a Spanish reformer writing in the eighteenth century of his countrymen's undiscerning awe of anything French, noted that if a French physician crossed the Pyrenees, Spaniards "thought they had gained a man capable of restoring souls from the other world."[83] The Spanish enthusiasm for foreign doctors was shared by the Mexican elite; their services were eagerly sought after by high society in colonial cities and some foreigners even married into powerful families.

The medical establishment, however, was inclined to view the situation differently. Foreigners tended to compete with Mexican practitioners in an area that hurt most: for the highest paying patients. Most Mexican médicos were creoles, a career in medicine offering them abundant opportunity for social prominence and financial reward. The increasing number of foreigners practicing medicine, especially in the eighteenth century—mostly French and English, but also Italian and Portuguese—provoked the local establishment to denounce the intruders frequently. The views of colonial officials were more ambivalent, however. On the one hand, the crown had mandated strict and copious laws regulating the entry of foreigners into the Spanish colonies. Any "prohibited person" wishing to reside legally in the Indies was required to undergo a lengthy and expensive process in which the applicant needed to accept the Catholic faith, obtain a special permit called *gracias al sacar,* be recognized as a proper emigrant by paying the *compuesto* to the *Casa de Contratacíon,* live continuously in the Spanish colonies for twenty years, hold real estate valued at 4,000 decats for ten years, and marry a native. In addition, those foreigners wishing to practice medicine had to hold a degree from a recognized university and then submit to the examination and licensing requirements of the Protomedicato. On the other hand, the authorities responsible for enforcing these laws often overlooked foreigners practicing medicine illegally in their jurisdiction.[84]

CURANDEROS

In the eyes of colonial authorities, the illegal practice of medicine had another component to it that went beyond the problems of licensing, one that bore more deeply into the heart of the colonial enterprise itself. All too often, medical beliefs transgressed into those of religion. The Church's formidable undertaking of eradicating idolatry and other "suspicious" practices meant that they would need to control the tide of healers that used incantations, spells, divination, or any form of sorcery to cure the sick. The overwhelming numbers of such healers doomed this endeavor from the start. Of course these practitioners, too, operated without a license, but it was the nature of the medicine they practiced that brought them to the attention of the authorities. Medical practices that violated church norms were investigated by the Inquisition if the perpetrators were Spaniards, blacks, or *castas*—people of mixed race. Indians, who remained outside the tribunal's jurisdiction, were subject to a parallel institution, the *Juzgado General de Indios,* founded in 1592, or the *Provisorato de naturales,* the tribunal for the archbishopric of Mexico that was charged with Indian affairs and oversaw matters of superstition, idolatry, witchcraft, and bigamy. Under the latter, it was common practice for local priests to gather information about suspect practices in Indian communities and, sometimes, to punish the perpetrators.[85]

Today, the word "curandero" brings to mind images of a healer working in long-forgotten traditions, dispensing herbal remedies, and curing curious ailments such as "evil eye" and "susto" by way of magic and ritual. But in the day-to-day world of colonial medicine, a curandero was not so clearly or narrowly defined. Sometimes it was simply the way licensed doctors described their unlicensed competition when denouncing them to the Protomedicato; often the lower-ranked practitioners were called curanderos as well. In early modern Spain the term was commonly used to refer to empirics of all kinds. Notary records of curanderos seeking licensees in sixteenth-century Valladolid give us an idea of the kinds of services they offered: listed are a Marcos de Castro, *sacamuelas*, or tooth-extractor; a Catalina de Castresana, specialist in "women's sickness"; an Alonso de Argüello, possessor of a secret powder to cure alcoholism *(contra el vino)*; Aparicio de Zubía, inventor of a medicinal oil; and María Hernández, *partera*, bonesetter, and applicator of "*bizmas*" (a type of plaster).[86] The word "curandero," then, like the term "cirujano," appears to have served as a sort of generic appellation for many types of empirically trained practitioners, a situation that conceals more than it illuminates for the historian interested in the marketplace of healers. In an effort to clarify the waters a bit, I limit my comments here to that spectrum of healers, both male and female, who utilized an assortment of indigenous, European, and African curing practices based primarily on manipulating supernatural forces. Although their methods of healing and skill level were as varied as their racial and cultural backgrounds, all of them combined magic and religion with some form of medical expertise.[87]

The colonial curandero's approach to medicine, whether practicing in Indian communities or in the more racially mixed Spanish towns, stood in sharp contrast to the university-educated physician, trained to see the human body in rational ways. The curandero was a specialist who claimed to have a unique intimacy with the supernatural elements of reality, a domain that was accorded an essential function by all cultures in New Spain, although to varying degrees. Serge Gruzinski makes the point that both the Europeans and the Indians "agreed in valuing the supernatural to the point of making it the ultimate, primordial and indisputable reality of things."[88] Of course, European notions of the supernatural, ostensibly controlled by the Church, differed radically from indigenous notions, both in concept and scope. The Church purposely restricted the domain of metaphysical reality by confining it to the Christian supernatural, while in effect excluding those states of being—drunkenness, dreams, hallucinations—to which indigenous cultures conferred a decisive significance because these states provided contact with divine entities and their powers.

But the task of the Church was further complicated by the fact that it did not hold a monopoly on Western forms of the supernatural. A multitude of individuals and low status groups from the Old World—conquistadores, farmers, artisans, African slaves, poor Spanish women—brought with them a mass of illicit beliefs and clandestine practices that the Tribunal of the Holy See sought to control. Colonial magic, whether originating from the Iberian countryside or African bush, differed from idolatry and Christianity in that it was not based on a body of doctrine meant to address the issues of human life; it offered no grand explanation of human existence, no promise of an afterlife. Its function was much more limited: it provided various remedies for illnesses, unhappy personal relationships, finding lost objects or animals, and protection from witchcraft. Lacking the guiding principles of religion, it was simply a collection of recipes, not a comprehensive view of the world. Emanating from a diversity of origins and uprooted from the environment that produced it, colonial magic mutated into a variety of modes, fusing indigenous, African, and European pagan practices into hybrid forms. Many of these were superimposed with Catholic ritual, distorting Christian prayers and invoking saints. In the unique environment of colonial Mexico, these disparate beliefs and practices were all set into motion, clashing and blending with one another, yet unified by a common objective: at a time when the state of medicine could offer the suffering and the diseased little real relief, the ritual of magic and contact with the supernatural provided a rich source of psychological support.[89]

How did one become a curandero? In many cases, induction into the profession came as a calling; in one manner or another, the healer was made aware of his or her healing powers and the obligation to use them. Sometimes this was revealed in a dream, or while enduring an illness. A near-death experience also could signal special healing powers; Ruiz de Alarcón mentions two indigenous curers who became aware of their calling through visions and dreams while gravely ill.[90] Just as in pre-Columbian times, certain people were considered to be more prone to having the "gift to heal"—*la gracia de curar*—or access to supernatural powers, especially those with physical defects. Jacinto de la Serna, writing about idolatry in the seventeenth century, noted that many of the indigenous curanderos he observed had some form of physical anomaly:

> . . . ugly old men and [those] marked by nature, or crippled or one-eyed, and their election to their priesthood or the gift *(gracia)* they have to cure, is attributed to those defects from which they suffer and the signals they have, and they say that when one lacks an eye or a leg, it gives them that gift.[91]

Those with a special calling to cure generally learned their craft under the tutelage of a practicing curandero. Not infrequently this apprenticeship took place within the confines of the family, the passing down of empirical know-how and rituals from one generation to the next. The craft of curing also could be learned with a specialist in the community, the would-be healer serving as helper and student concurrently. Some practitioners took on several apprentices at one time; in the late colonial period, both the mulata curandera Dominga Nuñez "La Polla," and the Indian Santos Bernabela had a group of young women under their instruction and supervision.[92]

Colonial curanderos differed radically from practitioners trained in humoral medicine in the ways they diagnosed the patient. The latter commonly viewed illness as the result of natural causes: body functions gone awry because of humoral imbalance, for example, or dietary mistakes, the effects of climate, even old age. Curanderos, by contrast, did not generally interpret sickness as an accidental phenomenon, but rather as "injury," a form of aggression perpetrated by some person (witchcraft) or supernatural entity (punishment). The tasks of the healer, then, were, first, to determine who or what was causing the harm—either a god, (or, by the seventeenth century, perhaps a saint), a sorcerer, or damage to one of the animistic entities in the body—and, second, to apply the appropriate treatment. The source of an illness might be discovered through the use—either by the patient or the practitioner—of psychotropics such as *peyote* or *ololiuhqui*,[93] whereas the treatment itself could entail any number of supernatural and empirical methods. Ritualized incantations, offerings, prayers, and confessions were common, as were such techniques as curing a wound with a curandero's breath, the painting of signs or figures (usually snakes) on the sufferer's back, head, or abdomen, or the sucking-out of various objects from different parts of the patient's body. In the latter case, illness could manifest itself in the most bizarre forms: Inquisitional documents show that curanderos extracted such things as insects and worms, strangely colored human and animal hairs, or small sticks and stones. These peculiar objects could be sucked out—the curandero used his or her mouth to do this—of any part of a patient's body, but most common was from the navel or somewhere on the face.[94] The healing methods of the indigenous curandero, at least during the first hundred years of the colonial period, had changed very little since the days of their ancestors.

An *Edicto de Fe* disseminated by the Provisor and Inquisitor of the Indies in 1796 indicates the kind of curing techniques the authorities deemed intolerable: "abuse of *pipilzitzintles*, *peyote* (both hallucinogenics), *chupamirtos* (hummingbirds), or roses, or other herbs, or animals; or feigning miracles, revelations, ecstasies, or raptures occurring to others so they may know things in the future, distant, or hidden, or executing them themselves; or carrying food offerings, figures, wax or incense to caves, hills, springs, ponds, or rivers, with the purpose of making offers to the air or other elements . . ."[95] In addition, the *inquisidores* were always watchful for practitioners who used language and ritual that, in the eyes of colonial authorities, transgressed official Christian doctrine. The ritualized use of prayers and orations by the laity strayed too easily into the realm of magic and pacts with the Devil. In 1784, José Antonio Hernández, a Spaniard, was arrested on charges of *curandero supersticioso*. Specifically, the Inquisition accused him of being a cheat and a liar *(engañador y embustero)*, who abused sacred things like the Holy Cross, benedictions and orations, pretending to see holy visions in the water, and having a pact with the Devil.[96] Hernández spent four years in the secret prisons of the tribunal while his case was being investigated and, in addition, his personal goods were confiscated to pay the cost of his stay. His story is typical of the individuals detained by the

Inquisition; stays were long, sometimes stretching into a decade or more, conditions were deplorable, and people often died while waiting for a verdict, as happened to the curandera María Tiburcia "La Gachupina."[97]

Awaiting the outcome of the investigation was often times worst than the final sentence. Curanderos, unless their crimes involved something more serious, for example, heresy, rarely were punished with life sentences, the most common penalty being a reprimand, which might be done privately or before the public. The guilty also were warned not to repeat their erroneous practices, as the inquisitors would not be so lenient the next time around. The patients who sought out these questionable cures were sometimes punished as well, their crime consisting in holding beliefs that offended the Catholic faith.[98]

Because most historical documentation on colonial curanderos centers around people being accused of superstitious practices and magic our view of them tends to be skewed. We are inclined to liken them to witchdoctors and shamans. But the repertoire of the curandero did not belong exclusively to the realm of the supernatural; most healers combined these practices with the standard therapeutic techniques of the day, such as bloodletting, purging, bathing, and massage. In addition, many of them had ample knowledge of Spanish and Mexican phamacopia. Ruiz de Alarcón describes several of the empirical remedies still being used in the seventeenth century, although without much interest, as the focus of his attention are the idolatrous incantations which always accompanied the cures. For broken bones, a plaster is made from an herb called *poztecpali,* which means "medicine for breaks." For stomach pain, a plant called *atliman,* is administered by means of an enema, and the "curing of diverse illnesses and pains" is treated by pricking the affected part with a needle or viper tooth. An innovative method of applying heat and pressure to a body in pain, called *tetleiccaliztli,* is worth describing is some detail:

> It is the case, then, that when someone is overly tired from walking or work or gets a chill while he is sweating from the excess of work or heat, and his spine has become stiff and taut, with pain in the loins, which also accompanies these troubles, in such a case these false doctors apply the cure that they call *tetleiccaliztli,* all of which consists in imparting warmth to the pained part with pressure, warming first a rock or comal. Then they stretch the patient face downwards on the floor, with all the back naked; then the false doctor with the staff in his hand thoroughly wets one foot, the calluses of which are like the knees of a camel because of excessive use. With the foot being thus wet, he places it on the very hot bowl or rock. He leaves it there until the heat penetrates the calluses to the live flesh. As soon as he feels that the heat has penetrated, he settles the foot, which is thus very hot, on the loins and spine of the patient, and when he presses down, the pain abates.

The pressure is applied while the curandero recites an incantation that summons the fire to aid him in combating the pain of the patient. The object of Ruiz de Alarcón's scorn however is not the physical technique, as "experience has well proved that those who suffer body pain . . . feel relief when their body is pressed on," but the "false and superstitious doctors" who have "introduced a deception with their excommunicated spells, attributing to words that which the act brings by itself."[99]

Indigenous curanderos were not the only ones to cure with words. In early modern Spain the function of the *ensalmador* was "to cure, with words of supplication and rare ceremonies, certain aliments in men and beasts."[100] In colonial Mexico, the inquisitors filled their secret jails with people whose curing methods inappropriately used the sacred rituals and images of the Catholic faith. A previously mentioned curandera, a mestiza called *la Gachupina*, working in Tepeji del Río in the late eighteenth century used prayers and orations to solicit the help of Jesus, the Virgin of Guadalupe, and San Antonio de Padua among others when applying herbal remedies. The Spaniard, Francisco Moreno, who practiced during the seventeenth century in Veracruz, Puebla, and Oaxaca, was arrested by the Holy Tribunal for "*curar ensalmos*." Brandishing a cross made from green sticks soaked in vinegar, water, or wine, he recited long orations invoking the help of Christ and the Virgin, a technique he claimed was especially useful in curing "wounds, ulcers, and apostems."[101] *Ensalmadores* dispensed specific orations for all sorts of maladies; there were those which stopped the flow of blood "from the nose or of women or of wounds," and those that cured "any wound, or ulcer or pain or any sickness." Curanderos promoted various orations as preventative medicine as well. One of these, recorded in the records of the Inquisition from the seventeenth century, promises that whomever carries with them the oration found in Holy Sepulcher of Our Lord Jesus Christ in Jerusalem, "will not die in prison, nor in battle, nor will they have epilepsy . . . nor will they die suddenly, not in fire, nor water, nor will they be faint of heart, nor bewitched, and if [the possessor] is a woman, she will have peace with her husband."[102]

Which social groups in New Spain consulted the kinds of curanderos I have been describing here? It seems that their services were in high demand at all levels of colonial society. Of course, the indigenous communities, especially those whose contact with the Hispanic world was limited, would have retained their medical culture long after the arrival of Europeans. But the colonial curanderos, at least those that operated within the gaze of the Church, practiced a medicine that has sometimes been described by modern researchers as *medicina mestiza*—medicine of the *casta* groups that had their origins in the conquest and whose numbers began to swell in the eighteenth century. It is within their ranks that we see the largest number of cases, the largest number of patients and practitioners alike, coming before the Inquisition.[103] True, this tribunal did not necessarily prosecute Indians, so many would not show up here; but we must keep in mind that the paucity of legally sanctioned practitioners throughout the colony made tolerance for indigenous healers a fact of life. The Spanish and creole groups of New Spain also sought out the specialized services of curanderos. One scholar, in fact, found that the bulk of patients cropping up in her study came from the Hispanic groups.[104] This is not surprising when we remember that Spanish popular medicine, although not approved of by university trained practitioners, was still very much a part of everyday life for most people. Indigenous practices penetrated this popular form of Western medicine, eventually crystallizing into a Mexican popular medicine whose traces are still seen today in many parts of the country. For people in colonial times, rational medicine could not offer superior services; thus, sufferers sought relief for their maladies from a variety of medical systems, with much less thought to ideological consistency than modern patients do.

THE CHURCH AND DIVINE HEALERS

Any exploration of the medical marketplace in New Spain would be remiss if it failed to mention the Church's role in providing medical care. Charity was an important element of Christian doctrine, and caring for the sick was one of the seven Works of Mercy outlined in the Gospel. In medieval Europe, ecclesiastics, especially those belonging to monastic orders, were important providers of charitable care for the sick and poor, mostly through institutions set up to offer food, lodging, and care for travelers and most varieties of the infirm and destitute. These early hospitals stressed hospitality rather than medical care and were commonly established on roads leading to shrines and cities. The monasteries also were instrumental in keeping ancient medical knowledge alive; their libraries housed the ancient manuscripts, and many monks who attended the sick had read the classic medical texts, blending them with popular remedies and spiritual healing. With the expanding urban economy of the High Middle Ages, and the corresponding reemergence of lay medical professions, the tradition of *medicina clericalis* began increasingly to confine itself to the charitable treatment of the poor and those beyond the reach of town-based practitioners.[105]

As organized providers of charity, it was natural that priests and lay members of the Church would have had a considerable role in tending the sick in Mexico. Throughout the colonial period, various individual members of religious orders practiced medicine in addition to their religious duties, especially in those parts of the colony where doctors were scarce or nonexistent, such as the north. Priests were part of the literate minority and most had the advantage of a broader education through which they would have had some exposure to the theories of medicine. In his much-cited essay about sixteenth-century doctors, Icazbalceta mentions two Franciscans lay brothers who practiced medicine, one in a convent in Mexico City, the other in Zapotitlán. The former, Fray Lucas de Almodóvar, was so well respected for his healing abilities that Viceroy Antonio de Mendoza, "fed up with the doctors," placed himself under the Brother's care and was completely cured.[106] It is also interesting to note that many of the first medical books published in early colonial Mexico were written by doctors and surgeons who later entered into religious life. Fray Agustín Farfan, whose book, *Tratado breve de Medicina*, was so successful that it was reprinted three times between the years 1592 and 1610, joined the Augustinian order after the death of his wife in 1568. The author of *Suma y Recopilatón de Cirugía*, Alonso López de Hinojosos, solicited to enter the order of The Company of Jesus in the last years of his life. From convents other authors, although not trained as doctors, wrote home medical guides for the layman, some that became standards of the time, such as Gregorio Lopez's *El tesoro de medicinias* and Juan de Esteyneffer's *Florilegio Medicinal*. The tradition of *medicina clericalis* remained strong in New Spain for obvious reasons: the existence of a large, poor, and suffering population underserved by legally trained medical attendants.

Hospitals were another way that the Church involved itself in medicine. Although a vigorous hospital movement had existed in Spain since the fourteenth century, during the reign of the Catholic Monarchs this escalated into a veritable boom, especially in those cities recently conquered from the Moors, such as Granada and Valencia. Hospitals were viewed by Church and Crown alike as an important tool in conversion and salvation. "Charity in the hospitals is extended to the Moor, to the Jew, to the heretic and gentile, and many are therein converted to the true faith of Jesus Christ," wrote a contemporary observer.[107] A few years later Pedro de Gante, one of the original twelve Franciscans to arrive in newly conquered Mexico, would make the same observation about the conversion of the Indians.[108] The Church's evangelical agenda coalesced perfectly with a royal agenda that sought to channel an ever-dwindling native population into productive enterprises, such as agriculture and textile production. Hospitals, along with the churches and monasteries linked to them, became important mechanisms through which the Spanish crown could attempt to aggregate a dispersed native population and achieve some degree of political, economic, and social control over them. Clearly, then, dispensing medical care was not the only motive here: political and economic goals merged with religious and humanistic ones in the founding of hospitals in New Spain.[109]

The mendicant orders were the first religious to found and organize hospitals in New Spain. In addition to their utility in the immense evangelical effort begun shortly after the conquest, hospitals were needed, it was argued, to assist and nurse the thousands suffering from the devastating epidemics that plagued Mexico during the sixteenth century. In 1555, the First Mexican Provincial Council mandated that each town should erect a hospital next the church, so that priests could easily visit the poor and sick to administer the sacraments.[110] The Augustinians and, even more so, the Franciscans distinguished themselves in the establishment of hospitals. In addition, a hospital association founded in the 1560s under the auspices of the order of *La Caridad y San Hipólito*, founded many hospitals throughout central Mexico. In 1589, they opened the Hospital of San Hipólito, the first institution dedicated to the treatment of the mentally ill in the Western Hemisphere.[111] Other early hospitals were founded by the Crown and prominent individuals. The Hospital Real de Indios, originally established by Pedro de Gante in the early 1530s, was later expanded and rebuilt by royal authorities to care exclusively for Indians. A large hospital for its time, its eight wards could accommodate more than two hundred sick and destitute Indians. And in 1521 Hernando Cortés established, and personally financed, the Hospital de la Concepción de Nuestra Señora, the first general hospital in New Spain, designed to care for the sick poor, both Spaniards and Indians; it excluded, however, patients suffering from leprosy, syphilis, madness, and St. Anthony's fire. The pueblo-hospitals established by Vasco Quiroga deserve special mention. Influenced by Thomas Moore's *Utopia*, he established pueblos in Michoacán where native Mexicans could be educated, converted, and protected from the abuses of Spaniards. Each community included a hospital containing separate facilities for patients with contagious diseases and was served by a physician, surgeon, and pharmacist. By the early seventeenth century, then, Mexico had a sizable network of approximately 128 hospitals, scattered throughout the most densely populated areas and along major roads.[112]

Two types of hospitals were established in New Spain: general and specialized. In cities, general hospitals—for example, Cotés's, which was built in the capital—were almost always located near the central plaza and the church. In 1573, a royal decree stated that "when a city, village, or place be founded, the hospitals for the non-contagious sick are to be placed next to the church, and for the contagious sick, erected in an elevated place where no ill winds passing through the hospitals are going to hurt the population." Colonial officials, no doubt, were motivated by the frequent epidemics and the contemporary notion that miasma, or bad air, caused disease.[113] Specialized hospitals, generally erected outside city environs, usually housed patients suffering from contagious diseases: leprosy, syphilis, insanity (which was thought to be contagious), and various forms of pestilence. Cortés built a leprosarium, the Hospital de San Lázaro, named for the patron saint of lepers, in Tlaxpana, outside Mexico City. Victims of syphilis, a widespread and virulent disease in the sixteenth century, were cared for at the Hospital del Amor de Dios, founded by Bishop Juan de Zumárraga in 1539.

How effective were hospitals at this time? Did they have any real impact on the state of public health? A realistic assessment of the early modern hospital demands first that we leave our current notions of this institution behind. The hospital, at the beginning of the twenty-first century, is central to modern medicine; it is where the most invasive and life-saving procedures are carried out, and where the elite members of the medical profession train, practice, and accrue status. It is also that part of medicine today that consumes the largest portion of health care budgets, at least in the West. But hospitals have not always been so essential to the practice of medicine, their centrality dating back only to the nineteenth and twentieth centuries. Before that they were simply one small part of the larger web of medical care, formal or informal. Early hospitals tended to be too few in number, restricted to certain social groups, employed too few medical staff, and had too little resources to be truly effective medical care providers.[114] Although colonial Mexico had an impressive network of hospitals, their overall effect on the population was probably more social than medical. They were helpful in reversing the dispersal of a native population overwhelmed by ravaging disease and the harsh treatment of *encomenderos*. Many of them, especially the pueblos, attracted Indians not only during times of epidemics and famine but also as residents of permanent status. They also functioned, as their founders intended, as centers for Spanish acculturation, with inhabitants learning not only the tenets of Christianity, but a new language and European medical ideas as well.[115] And equally important in a rugged and vast land such as Mexico, colonial hospitals provide a sanctuary for travelers and passers-by; one sixteenth-century observer described these retreats as a places where "travelers are entertained, and the sacraments of penitence and supreme unction are administered."[116]

The hospitals had both positive and negative effects on the health of its patients. Contagious disease was probably spread by assembling the infectious in one location, especially since isolation procedures were then largely ineffective. Perhaps the removal of the sick from the remaining population helped check the spread of disease somewhat, but this is not known. However, the comfort and health benefits of the nursing provided by the hospital staff—that is, the furnishing of food, water, rest, and clean, warm clothing—undoubtedly saved many lives. The hospitals of New Spain also occasionally contributed to the study of medicine by providing patient populations on which native medicines were used. The physicians at the Hospital de Santa Cruz in Huaxtepec, for example, experimented with many native plants to treat a variety of illness, including syphilis. Francisco Hernández, the well-known protomédico who came to New Spain to study native medicines, learned a great deal about medicinal plants at this hospital and returned to the capital with a rich harvest of information.

Autopsies also were sometimes performed on deceased patients, furthering the study of anatomy and pathology.[117]

And what of the other type of healing, the "divine" medicine of Christ, mediated through a variety of earthly representations of virgins, the saints, and Christ himself? In addition to the hospital, the Catholic Church in New Spain offered and encouraged a number of other healing rituals which fortified its position in colonial society. By the end of the sixteenth and beginning of the seventeenth centuries, it had disseminated an enormous quantity of prayers, novenas, and religious tracts for the prevention and cure of disease. These little booklets, with their novenas to an infinite number of medically specialized saints—to San Roque for protection against pestilence, for example, or to San Rafael for protection during childbirth—were reprinted by the thousands and provided another form of medical treatment when "earthly" medicine failed.[118] Catholic public ritual also promoted a cult of saints with healing powers. Processions through the streets must have been a common sight in most cities and towns, especially during times of pestilence and drought, and chronicles of the time are filled with notices of them. In January 1737, *procesiones y novenarios* to various divine images were made through the streets of Mexico City "to ask for relief from the fiery epidemic that people are suffering from in this kingdom." Several months earlier, a pestilence of *matlazáhuatl* had killed more than six thousand people in Puebla; after a procession and novena was made to the image of Jesus of Nazareth, "the number of sick diminished." And in the summer of 1735, when no rains had yet come, Church officials began a *novenario* to the Virgin de los Remedios "to appeal for the health of the public and speedy rains for relief from the suffocating heat, the cause of so many illnesses."[119]

The accounts of miraculous healing that circulated throughout New Spain highlight a clearly defined "hierarchy of resort," in which healing saints stood alongside domestic remedies and local medical practitioners. Reliance on divine intervention through the different avocations of the Virgin Mary and Christ, or popular saints was in large part a sign of desperation; only when earthly measures had failed was a direct appeal for a miracle in order. By the end of the first century of Spanish rule, miraculous images and their shrines were to be found all over the colony, from the northern frontier to the southern reaches of what today is Guatemala.

The Mexican cult of healing saints has its origins in the tradition of pilgrimage practiced in medieval Europe. Saints as healers did most of their work after death, that is, through direct contact with their relics, or physical remains, or with the tomb that held them. People believed that healing could occur through direct contact with the relics—by touching them, drinking water or wine in which they had been dipped, sleeping next to the tomb, or eating dirt scraped from the site. Seeking this kind of medical help then almost always involved a pilgrimage to a shrine, an expensive, inconvenient, and time-consuming endeavor in a time when travel was dangerous and difficult, and most Europeans were desperately poor. This also meant that the kinds of maladies that sent sufferers on such a journey were mostly of a chronic or congenital nature; the acutely ill undoubtedly sought care from local practitioners, and had either died or recovered before deciding to take to the road. Sometime in the fourteenth century, this pattern of faith healing began to change. It became more common to hear of miracles occurring without direct contact with relics, mediated instead by an image of the saint or by a vision or prayer. It was at this time, too, that Christians began to make pilgrimages after the miracle they had requested materialized, rather than before. This change in religious practice held significant implications for miraculous healing: if saints could heal at a distance, then sufferers of acute illness could invoke them as well as those suffering from chronic disease. Furthermore, saints—or rather the custodians of their shrines who lived off its proceeds—could begin to specialize in curing specific diseases, without reducing the pool of potential patients. Indeed, specialization had a definite appeal to patients who wanted to feel that they had placed their illness in the most capable hands. It is in this way that many saints came to be identified with specific diseases: St. Sebastian with plague, for example, St John with epilepsy, and St. Maur with gout.[120]

The New World, of course, did not possess many Christian saints and the relics that did find their way to the Americas generally remained in cathedrals and monasteries, where they were reserved for the contemplation of the elite. Yet the mass evangelization initiated by the Catholic Church generated a need for objects of popular devotion. In Mexico, this need was met not by saints' relics, but by sacred images of Christ and the Virgin, many of them miraculously appearing on spots previously considered sacred by precontact inhabitants. Over the years, thanks to an oral tradition of legends and testimony of divine interventions and miracle cures, these images became objects of votive supplication.[121] The most vivid historical evidence of this spiritual medical marketplace exists in the ex-votos from the colonial period and nineteenth century. Although we explore them in more detail in Chapter 5, this is an appropriate place to let one of them illustrate the kind of specialized healing for which the divine images of Mexico were well known. The sufferer is Don Luis de Isetaniux, a resident of Mexico City in the year 1799. He is ailing from "suffocation of the chest, an inflammation of the blood, and gushing blood from the mouth; and according to the doctors [. . .] little chance of survival." He implores the Christ figure—in this case, unnamed—for "the favor of being completely cured," which apparently occurs, and for which "this retablo is offered to give him thanks."

The cult of healer saints was just one more option, albeit one of last resort, in the vast and heterogeneous medical marketplace that flourished in New Spain.

As we have seen, when a medical practitioner is defined as anyone who appeared to sufferers themselves as medically skilled and experienced, than the variety of legitimate healers operating in this colonial world was quite extensive. This diversity is understandable when we consider that religious interpretation—both Christian and indigenous—was still an important way of making sense of everyday life, including health and illness. Likewise the state of contemporary medicine was such that no single group of practitioners could claim greater success than others; the physician, with all his years of book learning, did not yet have unique access to an esoteric knowledge, as his modern counterparts would later in the twentieth century. The polarities we would expect to draw as ways of distinguishing medical traditions—professional versus lay, literate versus oral, secular versus spiritual—only began to take shape in late colonial Mexico, and even then, only in the cities.

Now that we have examined some of the central circumstances surrounding human health in colonial Mexico—what people suffered from, and from whom they might have sought medical help—we turn our attention to the ways in which people understood how and why they became sick. This exploration takes several paths. We begin with a look at Mesoamerican etiology, that is, the conceptual framework precontact Mexicans used to explain their illnesses, an essential starting point for understanding indigenous health concepts in the colonial period. Next, we explore European explanations for illness and ideas on health maintenance, specifically those concepts based on humoralism, which looked to the environment and lifestyle as sources of illness. And, finally, our survey of everyday health experience ends with a closer look at how concerns about being sick textured daily life, including the role religion played in shaping the encounter with illness.

NOTES

1. Roy Porter, *The Greatest Benefit to Mankind: A Medical History of Humanity* (New York: W.W. Norton & Company, 1997), p. 31.

2. Margaret Pelling and Charles Webster, "Medical Practitioners," in *Health, Medicine, and Mortality in the Sixteenth Century*, ed. Charles Webster (Cambridge: Cambridge University Press, 1979), p. 166.

3. Margaret Pelling, *The Common Lot: Sickness, Medical Occupations and the Urban Poor in Early Modern England* (London: Longman, 1998), p. 1.

4. *The Badianus Manuscript*, intro., trans., and annotations by Emily Walcott Emmart, (Baltimore: Johns Hopkins University Press, 1940); Francisco Hernández, *Histo-*

ria Natural de la Nueva España, 2 vols. (México: UNAM, 1959). Two recent outstanding books in English have given new attention to Francisco Hernández's work and its dissemination in early modern Europe: Simon Varey, ed., *The Mexican Treasury: The Writings of Dr. Francisco Hernández*, trans. Rafael Chabrán, Cynthia L. Chamberlin, and Simon Varey (Stanford: Stanford University Press, 2000); and Simon Varey, Rafael Chabrán, and Dora B. Weiner, eds., *Searching for the Secrets of Nature: The Life and Works of Dr. Francisco Hernández* (Stanford: Stanford University Press, 2000).

5. Hernando Ruiz de Alarcón, *Treatise on the Heathen Superstitions That Today Live Among the Indians Native to This New Spain, 1629*, trans and ed. J. Richard Andrews and Ross Hassig (Norman: University of Oklahoma Press, 1984).

6. Fray Bernardino de Sahagún, *Florentine Codex: General History of the Things of New Spain*, 13 vols., trans and ed. C. E. Dibble and A. J. O. Anderson (Salt Lake City: University of Utah Press, 1950–69); Fray Bernardino de Sahagún, *Historia general de las cosas de Nueva España*, 4 vols., ed. A. M. Garibay (México: Editorial Porrúa, 1956).

7. Bernard R. Ortiz de Montellano, *Aztec Medicine, Health and Nutrition* (New Brunswick, NJ: Rutgers University Press, 1994), pp. 16–20.

8. Carlos Viesca Treviño, "El médico mexica," in *México antiguo*, eds. Alfredo López Austin and Carlos Viesca Treviña, Vol. I. of *Historia general de la medicina en México*, gen. ed. Fernando Martinez Cortés (México: UNAM, Acadamia Nacional de Medicina, 1984), p. 217.

9. Aguierre Beltrán, *Medicina y magica: El proceso de aculturación en la estructura colonial*, 2nd ed. (México: Fondo de Cultura Económica, 1992), p. 49.

10. Alfred López Austin, "Sahagún's Work and the Medicine of the Ancient Nahuas: Possibilities for Study," in *Sixteenth-Century Mexico: The Work of Sahagún*, ed. Munro S. Edmonson (Albuquerque: University of New Mexico Press, 1974), pp. 205–24, esp. pp. 216–17.

11. Sahagún, *Historia general* , Vol. III, pp. 116–17; Viesca Treviño, "El médico mexica," p. 220.

12. Viesca Teviña, "El médico mexica," p. 219.

13. Ruiz de Alarcón, p. 143

14. Sahagún, *Historial general*, Vol. III, p. 129; Ruiz de Alacrón, pp. 143–55.

15. Viesca Teviña, "El médico mexica," p. 219.

16. Sahgún, *Historia general* , Vol. II, p. 169.

17. Ibid., Vol. III, p. 129

18. Viesca Teviña, "El médico mexica," p. 222.

19. Sahagún, *Historia general*, Vol. I, p. 47; Vol. II, pp. 177–8, 174, 178–9.

20. Ibid, Vol. II, pp. 169–83.

21. Viesca Treviña, "El médico mexica," p. 222–3.

22. Aguirre Beltrán, p. 46; Viesca Teviña, "El médico mexica," p. 225.

23. Alfredo López Austin, *The Human Body: Concepts of the Ancient Nahuas*, 2 vols., trans. Thelma Ortiz Montellano and Bernard Ortiz de Montellano (Salt Lake City: University of Utah Press, 1988), Vol. I, p. 206; Ruiz da Alarcón, pp. 161–67; Viesca Teviña, "El médico mexica," p. 224.

24. Ruiz de Alarcón, pp. 59–67.

25. Sahagún, Fray Bernardino de, *Florentine Codex*, X, pp. 139–63; Aguirre Beltrán, p. 46; Viesca Treviña, "El médico mexica,"p. 223.

26. Viesca Treviña, "El médico mexica," p. 230; Sahagún, *Historia general* . . . , Vol. III. pp. 113–116.

27. Sahagún, *Florentine Codex*, X, p. 30.

28. Sahagún, *Historia general* . . . , Vol. III, p. 117.

29. For more on the bureaucratic oversight of the medical profession in sixteenth-century Spain, see Michele Lee Clouse, "Administering and Administrating Medicine: Regulation of the Medical Marketplace in Philip II's Spain" (Ph.D. diss., University of California, Davis, 2004).

30. John Tate Lanning, *The Royal Protomedicato* (Durham, NC: Duke University Press, 1985), p. 16.

31. Ibid., p. 21.

32. Ibid., p.48.

33. John Jay Tepaske, "Regulation of Medical Practitioners in the Age of Fancisco Hernández," in Varey et al., eds., *Searching for Secrets of Nature*, pp. 55–8.

34. Lanning, *The Royal Protomedicato*, p. 143.

35. Luz María Hernández Sáenz, *Learning to Heal: The Medical Profession in Colonial Mexico, 1769–1831* (New York: Peter Lang, 1997), p. 21.

36. Guenter B. Risse, "Medicine in New Spain," in *Medicine in the New World: New Spain, New France, and New England*, ed. Ronald L. Numbers (Knoxville: University of Tennessee Press, 1987), p. 37.

37. See John Tate Lanning, *Pedro de la Torre: Doctor to Conquerors* (Baton Rouge: Louisiana State University Press, 1974).

38. Lanning, *The Royal Protomedicato*, p. 139.

39. Risse, p. 14.

40. Lanning, *The Royal Protomedicato*, p. 182.

41. Ibid., pp. 331–2.

42. Bernal Díaz, pp. 356 and 565.

43. Dr. Francisco Fernandez del Castillo, *La cirugia mexicana en los siglos XVI y XVII*, (New York: E.R. Squibb & Sons, 1936), p. 3.

44. Lanning, *The Royal Protomedicato*, p. 261.

45. Ernestina Jiménez Olivares, *Los médicos en el Santo Oficio* (México: Departamento de Historia y Filosofia de la Medicina, 2000), pp. 17–19.

46. Francisco Fernández del Castillo, *La facultad de medicina: Segun el archivo de la Real y Pontífica Universidad de México* (México: Consejo de Humanidades, 1953), pp. 166–7.

47. See Clouse, especially ch. 3, "From Marketplace to the University: Creating Surgical Boundaries," pp. 102–141, on Philip II's regulations allowing empirics to seek licenses to practice their craft legitimately. Clouse's argument is that by legitimizing competent empirics, many of them were able to contribute their practical, hands-on experience to the theoretical development of medical knowledge.

48. Risse, pp. 22–4.; Ghislaine Lawrence, "Surgery (Traditional)," in CEHM , Vol. II, p. 969; Rafael Chabrán, "The Classical Tradition in Renaissance Spain and New

Trends in Philology, Medicine, and Materia Medica," in *Searching for the Secrets of Nature*, eds. Varey et al., pp. 23, 27–8.

49. Peter O'Malley Pierson, "Philip II: Imperial Obligations and Scientific Vision," in *Searching the Secrets of Nature*, ed. Varey et al., pp. 11–17. The economic explanation for Spain's limited contribution to scientific knowledge is made by David Goodman, *Power and Penury: Government, Technology, and Science in Philip II's Spain* (New York: Cambridge University Press, 1988).

50. Susan Lawrence, "Medical Education," in CEHM, Vol. II, p. 1164.

51. Hernández Sáenz, pp. 80–104.

52. Lanning, *The Royal Protomedicato*, p. 264–6.

53. Risse, p. 14.

54. Lannning, pp. 33–6.

55. Ibid., pp. 284–5.

56. Franciso Cervantes de Salazar, *México en 1554 y Túmulo imperial*, ed. Edmundo O'Gorman (México: Editorial Porrúa, 1972), p. 42.

57. José Sanfilippo Borrás, "La atención dental durante el virreinato," in *Temas medicos de la Nueva España*, ed. Enrique Cárdenas de la Peña (México: Instituto Cultural Domecq, A.C., 1992), p. 243; Lanning, *The Royal Protomedicato*, p. 285.

58. Lanning, *The Royal Protomedicato*, p. 285.

59. Hernández Sáenz, p. 195.

60. Sanfilippos Borrás, p. 244.

61. Fernandez del Castillo, *La cirugia mexicana en los siglos XVI y XVII*, pp. 9–10.

62. Hernández Sáenz, pp. 143–9; Paula De Vos, "The Art of Pharmacy in seventeenth- and eighteenth-century Mexico" (Ph.D. diss., University of California, Berkeley, 2001), pp. 28–9.

63. De Vos, pp. 32–3.

64. Lanning, *The Royal Protomedicato*, p. 231; DeVos, p. 25.

65. Hernández Sáenz, p. 151.

66. De Vos, pp. 392–8.

67. Hernández Sáenz, p. 150.

68. This lawsuit was brought to my attention by Paula DeVos, who graciously shared with me the documents pertaining to it. They can be found in: AGN/M Civil, L. 143, 2a Pte, Exp. 9/19, 1799. Paula also discusses this case in her dissertation on pp. 65–7, 241–58.

69. DeVos, pp. 39–44.

70. Fernandez del Castillo, *La facultad de medicina segun el archivo de la Real y Pontifica Universidad de México* (México: Consejo de Humanidades, 1953), pp. 191–201.

71. Robert MaCaa, "The Peopling of Nineteenth-Century Mexico: Critical Scrutiny of a Censured Century," *Statistical Abstract of Latin America*, ed. James W. Wilkie (Los Angeles: UCLA Latin American Center Publications, 1993), Vol. 30, part 1, p. 620.

72. AGN. Inquisición: 301.12 (1614); AGN. Inquisición: 873.12 (1777), cited in Gonzalo Aguirre Beltran, *Medicina y magica: el proceso de aculturación en la estructure colonial*, (México: Instituto Nacional Indigenista, 1963), pp. 337, 370. For a more recent

study that explores the linkages between female healers—including midwives—race, culture, and the Spanish colonial state in Guatemala, see Martha Few, *Women Who Live Evil Lives: Gender, Religion, and the Politics of Power in Colonial Guatemala* (Austin: University of Texas Press, 2002).

73. Adrian Wilson, "Participant or Patient? Seventeenth Century Childbirth from the mother's point of view," in Roy Porter, ed., *Patients and Practitioners: Lay Perceptions of Medicine in Pre-industrial Society* (Cambridge: Cambridge University Press, 1985), pp. 133–7.

74. Dr. Nicolas Leon, *La Obstetrica en México. Notas bibligráficas, étnicas, históricas, documentarias y críticas. De los orígenes históricos hasta el año 1910* (México: Tip. de la Vda. de F. Diaz de Leon, Sucrs, 1910), p. 120.

75. Ibid., pp. 101, 124, 142, 146–51.

76. Irvine S. L. Loudon, "Childbirth," in CEHM, Vol. II, pp. 1050–3.

77. Nicolas Leon, p. 323.

78. De Vos, p. 50.

79. Lanning, *The Royal Protomedicato*, p. 136; Carlos Viesca Treviño, "*Curanderismo* in Mexico and Guatemala: Its Historical Evolution from the Sixteenth to the Nineteenth Century," in *Mesoamerican Healers*, ed. Brad R. Huber and Alan R. Sandstrom (Austin: University of Texas Press, 2001), pp. 49–50.

80. De Vos, p. 50.

81. AGN, Protomedicato, III, Exp. 3. "Quejas del doctor don José Sánchez Camaño sobre los perjuicios que causan los curanderos que se consienten en el Valle de Santiago, intendencia de Santiago,"cited in John Tate Lanning, "The Illict Practice of Medicine in the Spanish Empire of American," in *Homenaje a Don José María de la Peña y Camara* (Madrid: Ediciones José Porrúa Turanzas, 1969), p. 161.

82. Archivo Historico de la Facultad de Medicina, "Causa criminal contra Nicolas Garica Miranda por haber curado a various sin ser facultativa," leg. 3, exp. 1, ff. 1–39, 1792, cited in Hernández Sáenz pp. 235–6.

83. Benito Gerónimo Feijóo y Montenegro, *Teatro crítico*, 2nd ed., 8 vols. (Madrid, 1773–81), I: 110; cited in Lanning, *The Royal Protomedicato*, p. 153.

84. Lanning, *The Royal Protomedicato*, pp. 153–68; Hernández Sáenz, pp. 54–63.

85. Nóemi Quezada, *Enfermedad y maleficio: el curandero in el México colonial* (México: UNAM, 1989), p. 107; Ruiz de Alarcón, p. 7; see also Serge Gruzinski's comments on sources and methodology in *The Conquest of Mexico*, pp. 305–8.

86. Anastasio Rojo Veja, *Enfermos y sanadores en el Castilla del Siglo XVI* (Valladolid: Universidad de Valladolid, 1993), p. 40.

87. Lanning, *The Royal Protomedicato*, p. 239; see also Viesca Treviño, "*Curanderismo* in Mexico and Guatemala," for a succinct introduction on curanderos in the colonial period.

88. Gruzinski, p. 184.

89. Ibid., 197–200; Luz María Hernández Sáenz and George M. Foster, "Curers and Their Cures in Colonial New Spain and Guatemala: The Spanish Component," in Huber and Sandstrom, p. 23; Keith Thomas, *Religion and the Decline of Magic* (New York: Charles Scribner's Sons, 1972), pp. 636–7; Aguirre Beltrán, pp. 75–112.

90. Ruiz de Alarcón, pp. 184–7.

91. Cited in Quezada, p. 36.

92. AGN, *Inquisición*, t. 1392, e. 22, ff. 357–71; AGN, *Inquisición*, t. 1433, e.25, ff. 215–24, cited in Quezada, pp. 39; Viesca Treviño, "*Curanderismo* in Mexico and Guatemala," pp. 58–60.

93. Ololiuhqui: psychotropic plant (Rivea corymbosa) whose active ingredients, the alkaloids D-lysergic and D-isolysergic acids, cause visions and "mystical" experiences in someone who ingests it.

94. Quezada, pp. 71–92; Hernández Sánez, p. 39; Ortiz de Montellano, pp. 162–81.

95. Cited in Quezada, pp. 109–10.

96. Ibid, p. 110.

97. AGN, *Inqusición*, t. 1300, exp. 12, ff. 175–364, cited in Quezada, p. 116.

98. Quezada, p. 117.

99. Ruiz de Alacrón, pp. 188–9, 189–90, 192, 183.

100. Marcelino Menendez y Pelayo, *Obras completas: historia de los heterodoxos españoles* (Madrid: Santander Aldus, S.A., 1946), Vol. I, p. 399, cited in Quezada, p. 101.

101. AGN, *Inquisicíon*: 478, exp. 83, ff. 510–15; *Inquisicíon* 1300, exp. 12, ff. 175–364; both cited in Quezada, pp. 102–4.

102. AGN, *Inquisición*, 283, exp. 3, f. 4: "Memoria de oraciones y ensalmos," *Inquisición*, 322, exp. 14, ff. 57–9, 364–7, 371–80, 386–90: "Oraciones recogidas por el Santo Oficio, una de ellas para contener las hemorragias"; *Inquisición*, 328, exp. 147, ff. 105–49: "Oraciones recogidas por la Inquisición contra la muerte súpita y contra todo mal," cited in Aguirre Beltrán, pp. 37–8.

103. See Aguirre Beltrán and Quezada's studies of curanderos in New Spain.

104. Quezada, pp. 121–2.

105. Colin Jones, "Charity Before *c.* 1850," in *CEHM*, Vol. II, pp. 1470–3.

106. Joaquín García Icazbalceta, *Bibliografía Mexicana del siglo XVI* (México: Fondo de Cultua Economia, 1954), p. 230.

107. Juan Santos, *Chronología Hospitalaria y Resumen Historial de la Sagrada Religion del Glorioso Patriarca San Juan de Dios*, 2 vols. (Madrid, 1715), Vol. I, p. 6, quoted in Risse, "Medicine in New Spain," p. 20.

108. Pedro de Gante to Charles V, October 21, 1532, in *Cartas de Indias* (Madrid,1877), no. 8, p.52, cited in Robert Ricard, *The Spiritual Conquest of Mexico* (Berkeley: University of California Press, 1966), trans. Lesley Byrd Simpson, p. 350.

109. Guenter B. Risse, "Shelter and Care for Natives and Colonists: Hospitals in Sixteenth-Century New Spain," in Varey et al., eds., pp. 66–8.

110. Ricard, p. 156.

111. See John S. Leiby, "San Hipólito's Treatment of the Mentally Ill in Mexico City, 1589–1650," *The Historian*, 54:1 (Spring 1992), 491–8.

112. Risse, "Medicine in New Spain," pp. 38–42; see also Guillermo Fajardo Ortiz, *Breve historia de los hospitales de la Ciudad de México* (México: Asociación Mexicana de Hospitales, A.C./Sociedad Mexicana de Historia y Filosofía de la Medicina, 1980); Josefina Muriel, *Hospitales de la Nueva España*, 2 vols. (México: Publicaciones del Instituto de Historia, 1956); Risse, "Shelter and Care," pp. 70–3.

113. Risse, "Medicine in New Spain," p. 38, royal decree can be found in Diego de Encinas, *Cedulario Indiano*, 4 vols. (1596; rpt. Madrid: Ed, Cultura Hispánica, 1945), Vol. I, folio 219, cited by Risse, p. 38.

114. Lindsay Granshaw, "The Hospital," in *CEHM*, Vol. II, p. 1180.

115. Risse, "Medicine in New Spain," p. 42.

116. Muñoz, Diego, O.F.M. "Descripción de la Provincia de los Apóstoles San Pedro y San Pablo en las Indias de la Nueva España," in *AIA*, Nov.–Dec. 1922, p. 399, cited in Ricard, pp. 157–8.

117. Risse, "Medicine in New Spain," p. 40 and 42.

118. Guerra, Francisco, "The Role of Religion in Spanish American Medicine," in *Medicine and Culture* (London: Wellcome Institute of the History of Medicine, 1969), p. 183.

119. *Gaceta de México*, "México," enero de 1737, t. I, no. 110, pp. 875–7; "Puebla de los Angeles," noveimbre de 1736, t. I, no. 74, p. 587; "México," septiembre de 1733, t. I, no. 70, p. 553.

120. Kathrine Park, "Medicine and society in medieval Europe," in *Medicine in Society: Historical Essays*, ed. Andrew Wear (Cambridge: Cambridge University Press, 1992), pp. 72–4.

121. Jorge Durand and Douglas S. Massey, *Miracles on the Border: Retablos of Mexican Migrants to the United States* (Tucson: University of Arizona Press, 1995), pp. 45–6.

3. THE WHOLE OF OUR FLESH

Our discussion of colonial healers in the previous chapter alluded to the variety of etiological beliefs that circulated throughout Mexico during the colonial period. All societies, be they small groups of hunter-gatherers, peasant-based systems, or industrialized societies, find a way to explain how and why people fall sick. Disease causes determine curing strategies. The treatment for an illness brought on by divine punishment, for example, will most likely incorporate the use of prayer and rituals of penitence, whereas an ailment caused by exposure to excessive cold may be treated with "hot" medicines and foods. Ideas about disease causation also tell us quite a lot about how people imagine the internal processes taking place in their otherwise opaque bodies. Even when causes were thought to originate outside the body, how did disease proceed once inside? What role did the blood and the vital organs play? Ultimately, agreed-on etiologies provide us with a window into a particular culture because they incorporate and confirm its basic ways of organizing the world. This is particularly apparent in the case of the Nahuas, whose worldview was constructed around the continual interplay between order and disorder, a process that had a profound effect on the welfare of human beings. Here, we look at native Mexican ideas about disease causation and, by extension, at conceptions about how the human body worked. Compared with contemporary European etiology, Nahua beliefs about how and why the body became ill are quite complex and defy easy categorization. Although both cultures perceived health threats along a continuum between natural and supernatural causes, native Mexicans accorded the supernatural much more involvement in human health than Spaniards did.

A SLIPPERY EARTH

Although it is impossible to convey the richness and breadth of the Mesoamerican worldview here, a brief overview is vital because ideas about health and disease were firmly grounded in underlying conceptions of how the world was structured. Human beings lived at the center of a universe where cosmic struggles acted themselves out in all aspects affecting human life. Although Mesoamericans and Europeans appeared to structure cosmic space in similar ways—the horizontal divisions of heaven, the underworld, and a terrestrial plane on which humans lived—this parallelism was superficial at best. One striking difference was the animate character of the Nahua universe; all features of their physical world—mountains, the wind, bodies of water, the sun, sky, and stars, as well as the earth itself—were animate beings.[1] In her astute work on the Christianization of Indians in the sixteenth century, Louise Burkhart notes that in such a world, so much of Nahua communication was directed toward interaction with nonhuman forces of nature rather than interaction with other human beings. Comparing this to a Christian cosmology which viewed the physical world as passive matter, she notes:

> When the very hills are alive, a people's place in the cosmos differs fundamentally from a world where human beings rule over a passive creation. The Nahuas did not set humanity off from the rest of nature like Christianity does. Human beings were part of the world; the world was not something to be rejected or striven against.[2]

Mesoamerican mapping of the universe placed the earth between a nine-layered underworld and a thirteen-layered heaven. This numerical division of space was linked to a parallel division of time. The 260-day ritual calendar was based on nine lunar months, the period of human gestation; when divided by twenty, the basic unit of the Mesoamerican number system, the result is thirteen. The calendar consisted of a repeating sequence of twenty day-signs, or *tonalli*, each paired with other repeating sequences corresponding back to the division of vertical space and day and night. Thus days, symbolically paired with the thirteen layers of heaven, occurred in units of thirteen; nights, corresponding to the nine layers of the underworld, came in units of nine. Each moment on earth, then, was influenced by a complex combination of phenomena originating in the various layers above and below the earth. The life of an individual was further influenced by his or her date of birth, or day-sign. One's *tonalli,* however, was not merely the imprint of a certain fate, but, rather, a kind of inherent animate force that had important effects on one's character and temperament. Specialists, the *tonalpouhque,* "enumerators of the tonalli," trained in reading the complex astrological influences of a particular day, were consulted to advise individuals on auspicious days for important events: the baptism of a child, the planting of crops, or the date of a marriage.[3]

Each level of the universe was associated with diverse gods and minor supernatural beings. Many of these deities were represented as conjugal pairs, reflecting the concept of cosmic duality, which was one of the key organizing factors in Nahua culture. Creation myths emphasized the male-female dichotomy—the prime creator gods were a male and female pair, Ometecuhtli, "Lord of Duality," and Omecihuatl, "Lady of Duality." Deities also exhibited contrary attributes within themselves. All goddesses of the earth-mother complex had some connection to fertility and death—for example, those in the myths surrounding Coatlicue, the great mother-goddess who gave birth to the sun, moon, and stars. Her son, Huitzilopochtli, the warlike god of the sun, killed and dismembered his siblings Coyolxauhqui, the moon goddess, and Centzon Huitznahua, a representation of the stars. Coatlicue thus embodied the dual concept of creation and destruction that the Nahuas saw as present in all life.[4]

Mesoamerican dualism was not merely an abstract philosophical principle but held sway over the everyday lives of individuals. Because gods contained opposite characteristics within themselves, particular deities could nurture crops and also destroy them, provoke sexual sin and forgive it, bring on illness and cure it. Other polarities helped to structure the natural world such as light and darkness, drought and humidity, hot and cold. These diametrical elements formed part of an overarching unity that could not be reduced to mere opposition between positive and negative; rather, each side formed an essential part of the whole. From death comes life, from destruction comes creation. The creative, positive forces and destructive, chaotic forces were two sides of the same coin, each dependent on the other for its functioning. In such a world, the primary challenge for human beings was to find the proper balance between order and chaos. Contact with chaos and disorder was essential because it was the source of life, yet one had to maintain the order and stability necessary for physical and social survival. As we will see, this order/disorder model significantly shaped ideas about moral conduct in everyday life and, in turn, about health. The association of sickness with disorder was a strong one in Nahua life; any form of sexual excess, immoderation in food or drink, any exposure to "filth" in both a physical and moral sense, could make one ill. These ever-shifting forces of order and disorder made the earth a particularly dangerous place. In quoting an adage recorded by Sahagún—"it is slippery, it is slick on the earth"—Burkhart notes:

> This was said of someone who had lived a good life but then fell into some *tlatlacolli* [wrong doing], as if slipping in the mud. It is easy to commit immoral acts not because demons tempt or the flesh is weak or the soul corrupt, but because of the nature of things: the earth is slippery.[5]

In such a precarious world, then, maintaining balance was essential. Keeping sickness at bay meant that one was continually working to preserve an equilibrium, not only in one's body, but in one's social relations and with the deities as well.

PICTURING THE BODY

According to Alfredo López Austin, the word the Nahuas used to designate the human body as a whole, *tonacayo*—literally, "the whole of our flesh"—was the same term used to refer to the fruits of the earth, especially maize, their most important food.[6] This metaphorical connection of physical sustenance with human flesh was not the only way Mesoamericans linked their corporal being to their cosmic structure. Like the natural world around them, human bodies contained several animate forces which were responsible for such things as development and growth, body heat, breathing, emotions and passions, and powers of perception. Three have been identified by scholars as being vital for the functioning of the body: *teyolia*, or *yolia*, located in the heart; *ihiyotl*, located in the liver; and *tonalli*, found in the head. Although the deities imbued humans with these forces, it seems that the Nahuas considered any change in them as essentially naturalistic in their effects on health. One way to understand this, for heuristic purposes at least, would be to distinguish between proximate and ultimate disease causes. Proximate, or natural, causes locate sickness as a result of routine bodily processes that have gone awry, the physical result of something tangible in the environment or a natural change in the condition of the individual. Thus, the effects of cold, heat, or fatigue, the consumption of certain foods or herbs, and the effects of old age would be viewed as proximate causes, just as would the injuries of the battlefield or work site, or an illness brought on by the bite of a poisonous snake. Ultimate causes, or theories about why such "natural" events happen in the first place, tend not to be found in natural phenomena or chance, but in what one scholar calls the "super-social relations of hostility," or the full extension of human society that includes supernatural actors.[7] Yet the disentanglement of natural from ultimate causes, although helpful to those of us who have a hard time envisioning bodily processes outside of a biomechanical model, is not something in which the Nahuas would have consciously engaged. Their view was much more holistic.

Like ourselves, the Nahuas conferred a central role to the heart in the human body. Not for its function of pumping blood, which we presume they did not know about, but because this was the location of the *teyolia*, the vital force responsible for one's knowledge, emotions, personality traits, and vitality. The *teyolia*, which was conveyed to the fetus during gestation, was a kind of divine force clearly seen in people of exceptional talent in the fields of religion and art. The good painter of codices, for example, was *yolteotl*, "deified heart," whereas the bad featherworker had a heart that was wrapped up, "his heart was covered." Damage to the heart brought on serious illness. The Nahuas believed some diseases covered the heart with phlegm. Molina, for example, refers to the expression *Tlayohuallotl mopan momana* as a loss of consciousness, or "an illness that envelops the heart and causes swooning." The *Relación de Yetecomac* refers to people who became ill because "their hearts were covered."[8] Many of the ailments mentioned in the *Florentine Codex* describe symptoms that involve the heart: a "nausea about the heart," an "anguished" heart, a "heart [that] seems faint," a "congested heart." *The Badianus Manuscript*, an indigenous herbal written in the mid-sixteenth century, recommends a strong purge for "oppression of the chest," an ailment that makes one feel "constricted" by a "certain fullness" in the chest area.[9]

Sixteenth-century friars chose the native *teyolia* or *yolia*, as a translation for *ánima*, or soul in their efforts to find parallels in native thought categories, although, as Burkhart points out, the frequent use of *ánima* alone in early religious texts suggests that they did not find the Nahua concept completely appropriate. Like the Christian soul, the *yolia* animated the body, was partly responsible for character, and survived after death; yet these similarities were more apparent than real. With its neat conception of the body/soul dichotomy, Christian theology separated the soul from the flesh in a way that the Nahuas never could; for them, the body was a composite of several fleshy and spiritual elements, all of which had to operate harmoniously for a person to maintain physical and mental health. Metaphysical elements of human existence were not set off from the material side of life, but were continuous with it, all integrated into a single monist conception of reality.[10]

Another important animistic force, *ihiyotl*, was found in the liver. It was closely associated with breath or respiration but also with passions and such feelings as anger and envy. There is some evidence to suggest that *ihiyotl* was thought to have qualities of a luminous gas which could influence other beings. The idea that emanations from one person, especially those who had committed immoral acts, could damage others was common among the Nahuas. Immorality was often expressed in terms of dirt or filth, *tlazolli*, with the offender becoming polluted and thus polluting to others. This contagious quality of pollution is the central idea underlying the concept of *tlazolmiquiztli*, "filth death" or *tlazolmiquiliztli*, "dying of filth." The filth resulting from transgressions lodged in the liver of the perpetuator, the seat of the *ihiyotl*; he or she, in turn, released emanations that were harmful to anything around them. Thus, a child could become ill by a parent's misdeed; turkey chicks died in the presence of someone involved in an illicit love affair; the emanations of adulterers could hurt their spouses; and merchants' goods could be damaged by their own sexual misdeeds.[11]

With *tlazolli* such a threat to well-being, it is not surprising to find that the symbolic manipulation of dirt and cleanliness constituted an important part of Mesoamerican ritual. The Nahuas' removal of filth centered on the rites of sweeping and bathing. According to Sahagún, homes and courtyards were swept daily, as indeed they still are today.[12] Sweeping, which removed polluting substances away from the center to the periphery where they belonged, was one of the penitential rites practiced on a daily basis.[13] *Tlazolli* affecting the body had to be removed by bathing. The infant was ritually bathed at birth to remove the "filthiness which thou has taken from thy mother, from thy father."[14] The *tlazolli* washed from the child was the residue of his or her parents' sexual activity, too much of which was thought to be harmful to the developing fetus. The elders who advised young pregnant women addressed the issue of sexual intercourse during pregnancy. In early stages of gestation, sexual activity was thought to be salutary because the accumulation of semen nourished and strengthened the fetus; later in the pregnancy, however, too much semen was a danger as it became sticky and viscous, increasing the baby's risk of becoming stuck during birth.[15] Removing the filth associated with sexual transgression frequently involved bathing. Ruiz de Alarcón identifies this as *tetlacolaltiloni*, a "bath for the sickness caused by love affairs or by affection," a ritual that, in addition to washing the body, involved special incantations and the use of incense.[16] Bathing was not solely tied to sexual violations; other crimes against the social order demanded a purification through washing as well. As they were being released from incarceration, prisoners who had been falsely accused or whose offenses had not been so grave, immediately bathed in the pure waters of Chapultepec "to lay aside their crimes." But to those who had committed more serious crimes—theft or adultery—the rebuke was unequivocal: "nowhere is there water with which thou wilt bathe thyself, with which thou wilt cleanse thyself."[17] Bathing was not always enough.

For the Nahuas, then, exposure to *tlazolli* had direct physical consequences. Filth and illness were so closely linked that Tlazolteotl, the goddess of filth was also the patron goddess of healers. Daily bathing with a soap made from the fruit of *copalxócotl* (cyrtocarpa educalis) was a common practice among the Nahuas, a custom that astounded the bathing-adversed Spaniards in the sixteenth century.[18] Moreover, the purifying effects of bathing were an important therapy in ancient Mesoamerican medicine. The healing properties of the *temazcal*, or sweat bath, still used today in some indigenous communities, presumably derived from its ability to induce sweating, ridding the body of *tlazolli* lodged in the flesh. According to the native doctors who contributed their medical knowledge to the *Florentine Codex*, this therapy was widely used to treat both physical and psychological symptoms:

> And the sick there restore their bodies, their nerves. Those who are as if faint with sickness are there calmed, strengthened. They are to drink one or another of the medicines, as has been mentioned. And one who perhaps has tripped and fallen, or who has fallen from a roof terrace; or someone has mistreated him—his nerves are shattered, he constantly goes paralyzed—they there make him hot. . . . And one who has scabs, [one] whose body is much festered, [one] whose body is not [too] much covered with sores, they there have [such as these] wash.[19]

Nahua notions of *tlazolli* vividly illustrate the strong links between the physical and the moral in Mesoamerican conceptions of the body, a link that was much more direct than it was for Europeans. Practices deemed as immoral were physically debilitating; failure to participate in penitential ritual could be punished with disease. Europeans, too, sometimes saw disease as punishment for sin, although this connection was more arbitrary than absolute. Rather, Christian doctrine tended to view this relationship in more symbolic terms. The condition of the body provides a metaphor for that of the soul; because the soul is immaterial, sickness can only be a metaphor for a soul corrupted by sin.[20] It was little wonder then that Spaniards and Nahuas had such different views of the body, health and illness, and even practices such as personal hygiene. Not sharing the same assumptions about illness and filth, early modern Europeans bathed infrequently and, in fact, thought that too much exposure to water was a threat to their health, a topic that we explore in Chapter 4.

The third animistic entity found in the human body was the *tonalli*, located in the head. According to Molina, this word was derived from the verb *tona*, "to irradiate," and had several meanings, including solar heat, summer, day, day-sign, one's destiny according to their birth date, and "soul or spirit." Many scholars have written about the nature of *tonalli*, from its ancient origins to its present-day permutations, and rightly so, as this multifaceted entity played—and in some indigenous groups still plays—a vital role in human life. An entire volume would be necessary just to examine its connection to the Mesoamerican calendar, day signs, human fate, and character. My goal here is more modest: to look at *tonalli* and its associations with sickness and health.

The idea of *tonalli* as a life force revolves around its role in giving the body its warmth. In some instances the Nahuas believed they could increase *tonalli* by placing the body next to a fire. According to Sahagún's informants, newborns were always placed by a fire for the first four days of their lives, after which time they would be ritually bathed and named. This fire was so vital to the infant's life that no one was allowed to light another from it as that would imperil the child's well being.[21] Physical growth was directly connected to one's *tonalli*, which would explain why the Nahuas attributed life force to body parts that grew, such as teeth, nails, and, especially, the hair. Because it was located in the head, a very close relationship existed between the *tonalli* and the hair. This gave rise to all sorts of beliefs about human hair: since it covered the head, protecting the *tonalli*, its removal could make a person vulnerable to illness; it was thought to have medicinal properties; it could exhibit a will of its own, like *tonalli* itself; and, because of its life-giving force, the hair of the deceased was kept in their memory. In addition, the hair of captives caught in battle could intensify the fighting powers of those who kept it, as could that of a woman who had died in her first childbirth. People performing tasks that demanded great energy and force could never cut or wash their hair. This was true of priests as well as traveling merchants who set out on long and arduous journeys.[22] Although the *tonalli* was found in the head, and cures associated with it were directed for the most part toward the crown of the head, the face, and forehead, its force flowed throughout the entire body. Just how the Nahuas thought this happened is not known, although indigenous groups today say the blood is its carrier. What is clear, however, is that ancient Nahuas thought *tonalli* was essential for life; the human body could live without it, but not for very long.

In his descriptions of indigenous healing methods in the seventeenth century, Hernando Ruiz de Alarcón describes how a female healer—known as *atlan tlachixque*, a "looker into water"—held a sick child over a pool of water in order to see its reflection. If the child's face was clearly visible, it had a good prognosis; if the face appeared dark, was difficult to see, "as if covered by some shadow," the child was judged to be suffering from a loss of *tonalli*, a potentially serious condition.[23] The Nahuas believed the *tonalli* left the body under certain conditions, such as during sleep or in the state of drunkenness, but there were special circumstances under which its departure might be especially dangerous. In the highly moralistic world of the Nahuas, it comes as no surprise to find that many of these situations revolved around sexual activity. Early sexuality diminished the *tonalli* and shortened one's lifespan, but even well into adulthood, a man was advised to be moderate, even with his own wife. "Thou art not to devour, to gulp down the carnal life as if thou wert a dog," the Nahua elders warned the next generation of young men. Immoderate sexual activity will drain a man of his strength, cause him to become dry and shriveled like a maguey plant from which the juice has been drained or a cape that has been washed and tightly wrung so that it dries quickly. "Not only art thou useless, but soon thy nasal mucus goeth hanging: thou wilt go toothless, thou wilt go on hand and knees, thou wilt go pale." In short, too much sex could make one sick. It is interesting to note, however, that the Nahuas did not appear to believe that women were as vulnerable to these dangers. Perhaps it was simply the case that women, being confined to hearth and home, did not need to be admonished as much as men. Yet the concern with men depleting their vital forces too early in life may also have had something to do with what happened during sexual intercourse itself: namely, that women did not suffer the fluid loss, through ejaculation, that men did. Sahagún's informants recount a short anecdote about older women seeking out younger men for sexual favors. When asked to give their reasons for this outrageous act they said:

> Ye men, ye are sluggish, ye are depleted, ye have ruined yourselves impetuously. It is all gone. There is no more. There is nothing to be desired. But of this, we who are women, we are not the sluggish ones. In us is a cave, a gorge, whose only function is to await that which is given, whose only function is to receive. And of this, if thou hast become impotent, if thou no longer arousest anything, what other purpose wilt thou serve?[24]

Because the *tonalli* was thought to leave the body briefly during coitus, any interruption during the sexual act itself, might prevent its full return. Likewise, a sudden fright or shock allowed the *tonalli* to escape—a belief that has survived in the present form of the folk illness *susto*. Molina translated the word *netonalcaualtilizli* as "he who is frightened of something," but it literally translates as "the loss of *tonalli*."[25] To be frightened during sexual intercourse must have been especially ominous, even for a married couple entitled to sex since their animating forces might flee their bodies and leave them vulnerable to sickness. Sahagún's medical informants mention medicine used to treat diseases brought on by a fright during sex, effective even if the man's "body turns black . . . when already he loses flesh; even if he has been sick one year, or perhaps already four years, it is required." The loss of *tonalli* through sexual intercourse was also a factor in an ailing patient's recovery. Many of the medicines listed by Sahagún are used in treating people who have had a relapse because they apparently engaged in coitus while they were still in a weakened state.[26]

As we can see from this brief discussion of the *teyolia*, *ihiyotl*, and *tonalli*, the physical and supernatural were tied to human health in ways that are very difficult to unravel. These animating forces, so vital to physical and psychological functioning, affected well-being in concrete ways—the *tonalli's* connection to body temperature and growth, for instance—yet they also appear to have been conduits through which supernatural forces, usually triggered by sexual transgression, manifested themselves inside the body. Disease, as with other kinds of misfortune, ultimately originated in the dialectical interplay between human behavior and chastising gods, a topic that we turn to in the next section.

DEITIES AND DWELLERS OF DANGEROUS PLACES

Mesoamerican religion encompassed a bewildering variety of supernatural forms that contrasted sharply with Western conceptions of deity. Some of these forces were major gods, for example, Tezcatlipoca, Quetzalcoatl, or Tlaloc, but many others were simply their envoys and helpers, or other kinds of spirits who resided in the peripheral zones of the earth such as caves, lakes, streams, and forests. The deities themselves embodied order and disorder, sometimes deceiving humans, other times bestowing on them acts of kindness. Huitzilopochtli, was a "madman, a deceiver," but also just a "common man"; Tezcatlipoca was a creator of things, yet he could bring "all things down," he mocked and ridiculed men, but "bestowed riches" on them as well; Tláloc, the god of rain, was the provider of things essential to life—the trees, grasses, and maize—yet he was the cause of death, especially by way of drownings and lightening bolts.[27] This extensive divine entanglement with life on earth meant that human beings, in order to limit their exposure to misfortune, were continually engaged in a process of propitiation. Gods had to be appeased, the calendar of rituals carefully observed, and penitential exercises avidly performed. One had to conduct one's life carefully, being sure to follow the guidelines laid down by the ancestors, least one slip and fall into the abyss. Burkhart notes that early colonial Nahuatl texts are full of "torrent-and-precipice" tropes—tripping and stumbling, falling off precipices and into caves—that stand in as metaphors for, or actual results of, moral straying.[28] For the Nahuas, the physical state of their bodies was bound to the conduct of mercurial gods: any violation of a moral code or failure to observe vital rituals—the transgressing of significant boundaries—exposed one to the unpleasant repercussions of disease.

Tezcatlipoca was the Nahuas' principle god and most likely the ultimate cause of all ailments attributed to supernatural powers. A complex deity, he appeared under many guises—Titlacahuan, Moyocoyatzin, Yaotzin, among others—and was closely associated with the forces of disorder and chaos, dirt and filth.

A skunk's entrance into one's house was an ominous sign that Tezcatlipoca was about to unleash his wrath: its foul stench "entered into one," auguring death and destruction. Sahagún's informers were very explicit about the afflictions he was capable of causing: "he stoned [men] with plagues, which were great and grave—leprosy, pustules, knee swellings, cancers, the itch, hemorrhoids, piles, humors of the feet, and still other sicknesses." Some gods were associated with specific diseases. Skin and eye afflictions were the province of Xipe Totec, a god affiliated with the renewal of spring and a deity favored by the Zapotecs. He tormented people with "blisters, festering, pimples, eye pains, lice about the eyes, opacity, filling of the eyes with flesh, withering of the eyes, cataracts, glazing of the eyes." Sexual intercourse during a fast was punished by Macuilxochitl, one of the flower deities, who gave the offenders "as their merit, their lot," venereal afflictions. The Tlaloc complex of deities caused people to suffer maladies and mishaps that the Nahuas associated with water—not only drownings and lightning strikes but also afflictions that caused the body to swell with fluid, such as dropsy or gout.[29]

Threats to health lurked in other supernatural aspects of the natural world as well: *echecame* and the *tlaloque*, spirits of the wind and waters respectively, resided in the mountains, caves, and springs. Ruiz de Alarcón mentioned a group of spirits that lived in the forest, the *ohuican chaneque*, or "dwellers of dangerous places." Because these were points of contact with the underworld, they represented to the Nahuas zones of the periphery, places of danger. The person who ventured into these sites risked contracting gout, "of the feet or hands, or of anywhere on the body," a stiff neck, or paralysis in one of the limbs.[30] The Nahuas made much reference to center and periphery in their discourse. Their dwelling place on earth put them right at the center of the universe. The Mexica, the dominate partners in the Triple Alliance that ruled much of central Mexico on the eve of the conquest, centered themselves in the heart of Tenochtitlan, symbolized by the Great Temple. Cities, with tidy houses and swept streets, were places of order; the space outside of town was liminal and dangerous. At the local level, one's home represented the center as well, a microcosm of ordered space.[31] One of the adages recorded by Sahagún, *otimatoiavi, otimetepexiuj*, "thou hast cast thyself into the torrent . . . from the crag," is said of someone who has crossed into the periphery with his or her behavior, one "who has placed [themselves] in danger . . . who brings about that which is not good."[32] All unchecked behavior exposed one to a precarious outcome. Burkhart offers an anthropological perspective:

> Movement into and out of ordered space had powerful moral implications. The argument operates on this analogy: secure center is to dangerous periphery as moral conformity is to immorality. Internal metaphor equates immoral acts with movement

> into dangerous places. This metaphor is treated metonymically, such that the immoral person is actually described as someone who enters these places, as if the act of movement and the immoral deed belong to the same behavioral domain.[33]

Another place fraught with symbolic danger was the crossroads. Associated with uncontrolled female sexuality, sorcery, and the underworld, this was where the Cihuateteo, the women who had died in their first childbirth, came to haunt people and inflict illness on children. When someone had seizures or convulsions, when "one's mouth was twisted, one's face was contorted; one lacked use of a hand, one's feet were misshapen," it was said of them they were possessed by the Ciuapipiltin, the goddesses who dwelt at the crossroads.[34] But one did not necessarily have to leave home to be exposed to the dangers of the periphery; a violator of moral codes could still bring the periphery to themselves. Book Five of the *Florentine Codex* lists all the *tetzahuitl*, usually translated as "omens," that filled the Nahuas with apprehension. Anything that was unexpected or frightening was a *tetzahuitl*, "an anomaly, a rupture of harmony, a little bit of chaos slipping into ordered reality." The cry of a wild animal at night, a wail that sounded "as if a poor old woman wept," could signal an impending death for the person who heard it. Owls with their piercing screeches were particularly ominous. If one cried in the presence of a person already sick, "they said that now he would not issue forth; now we would take our leave of him."[35]

Sickness caused by the deities was treated with special prayers, rituals and offerings, acts of penitence, and confession. Those afflicted with the skin and eye diseases of Xipe Totec, for example, pledged to participate in his feast day celebrations by wearing the flayed skins of the victims that had been sacrificed at the beginning of the celebration. By wearing the flayed skins, then shedding them, they symbolically took part in the renewal of the "skin" of the earth.[36] People who committed grave offenses such as adultery could cleanse themselves by the rite of confession, although this was a once-in-a-lifetime opportunity. Confession was the province of the male/female deity pair, Tezcatlipoca and Tlazolteotl, the gods most associated with sexual violations. Together they had the power to cause sexual transgressions, punish the offenders, and remove the impurities—the *tlazolli*—that adhered to the perpetrator of such acts. Tlazolteotl, the "Filth Deity," governed the domain of "evil and perverseness, debauched living"; such were the things Tlazolteotl "offered one, cast upon one, inspired in one. And likewise she forgave one, set aside, removed [corruption]. She cleansed one; she washed one." In her guise of confessor, she became Tlaelquani, the "Filth Eater," because she ate the sins of her penitents, taking on their filth. After confessing to a human mediator—"the wise one, in whose hands lay the books, the paintings"—the penitents were then instructed to perform further rites such as fasting or passing reeds through their tongue, ear, or penis.[37] The Nahuas called this rite of confession *neyolmelahualiztli*, "straightening one's heart," a practice that restored internal equilibrium by returning the heart to its proper place. For the Nahuas this practice was directly linked to physical health. It is interesting to note that the early missionaries adopted this word as a term for the Christian rite of confession. Burkhart notes that in doing so, the friars

> not only fomented an identification, in form and function, between the Nahua and the Christian rite, thus aiding in the new rite's acceptance, but also implicitly accepted Nahua concepts of the body and its relationship to morality.

Many of the friars writing in the sixteenth century, such as Mendieta and Motolinía, commented on how well the Indians took to the Christian rite of confession. They confessed frequently, often bringing the sick and lame to confess. No doubt the natives' acceptance of this Christian sacrament had more to do with its perceived curative powers than with the spiritual act of penitence that the friars tried to convey.[38]

If deities and other supernatural forms could cause sickness through a bewildering variety of mechanisms, it is not surprising to find that human beings could also bring on illness in others. We have already seen that someone whose liver had taken on a great deal of *tlazolli* by his or her actions also might become infectious to others around them; this was the notion behind *tlazolmiquiztli*, or "filth death," whereby a parent might unintentionally infect her child with the filth that adheres to her from engaging in illicit sexual activity. But some people were capable of inflicting bodily harm in others intentionally. A common name for sorcerers was *tlacatecolotl*, "owl man," a person associated with the night and the underworld, someone who derived his powers from being born on an inauspicious day of the Mesoamerican calendar, such as 1-wind. It was said of such a person that he "had spells to cast . . . he was evil, corrupt, one who deluded, laid enchantments." Sorcerers could attack the body of their victims in a variety of ways: by causing the intrusion of objects—pieces of bone, stones, or sticks—into the body; by "squeezing," "whirling," or "eating" the hearts of their victims; or by attacking the calves of someone's leg so they would have cramps when they walked.[39]

Nahuas' bodies then were directly linked to the various supernatural forces operating in this multilayered cosmos. Volatile deities and their earthly envoys lurking in streams and caves punished uncontrolled behavior and ritual breaches with disease. Yet the language of offence and penance, which so thoroughly permeates sources like the *Florentine Codex*, at times puts forth a simplistic image of Mesoamerican religion—one of outraged gods punishing sinners for their disobedience—and can easily mask a more nuanced reading of

Nahua culture. People who committed social violations did not simply disobey rules laid down by divine authority; rather, they transgressed critical social boundaries, entering zones of disorder and chaos. Yet such was the nature of the world—its slipperiness, its danger. The Nahuas came to terms with this reality, not by rejecting it, but by trying to live within it. Their method was to foster a value system based on the virtues of moderation, a balancing act between order and chaos. Bodily equilibrium was central to this process.

FINDING EQUILIBRIUM

Jacques Soustelle noted long ago that two conflicting value systems dominated Aztec culture, that of the warrior ethic and the ideal of moderation and restraint.[40] The *Florentine Codex* makes this distinction quite clear: the "wicked but brave warriors, those furious in battle" paid their tribute in death, whereas it is "the weepers, the sighers, those who humbled themselves" who are destined to rule.[41] Burkhart dissects this even further; the fiercest and bravest warrior, she writes, "is not so much a moral ideal as a special-function anti-ideal—immorality for a purpose." The opposition in these two ideals parallels the opposition between order and chaos, both of which are inevitable and desirable. In the slippery world of the Nahuas, overindulgence and excess opened one up to all sorts of peripheral dangers, yet its complete absence brought sterility and stagnation; best was to pursue the middle way, to maintain an equilibrium as best as one could.[42]

These contrasting values were clearly reflected in Nahua concepts about the body, which depicted health as a state of equilibrium between the human body and the cosmic forces with which it was constantly interacting. Any alteration in the system might manifest itself in bodily changes, producing a loss of balance. This lack of equilibrium was often expressed by Nahua sources as an opposition—or, more accurately, a dialectical unity—between hot and cold, qualities that were applied to a whole range of beings and things in the world. Deities of the upperworld were of a hot nature, a quality reflected in their colors and their attire, while those of the underworld were cold. Human beings, centered as they were on the earth, were an amalgam of the two. The *tonalli*, along with its place of residence in the body, the head, was hot; the *ihiyotl*, and by extension the liver, was colder. Fatigue, brought on by hard work or prolonged walking, heated one up, whereas rest cooled one down; sexual arousal was hot, its gratification cooling. Nahuatl terms that describe activity and rest reflect a hot/cold polarity. The verbs *ceceltia* and *cehuia* mean "to rest" and "to cool what is hot," whereas *tonalcehuia*, "to rest one who walks," literally translates as "to cool down the *tonalli*."[43] Many of the medicines listed by Sahagún's informants were used to heat up or cool down the body. *Chichientic*, an herb with blossoms similar to the amaranth plant, was used for cooling the body after a purge, and a person suffering from diarrhea and fever was advised to eat only cooling foods along with a drink made from the *tlalmizquitl* root, which reduced the body's heat.[44] The *Badianus Codex* mentions illnesses that were caused by too much heat, notably those located in the heart, head, and eyes, and one in which coldness settled in the abdomen. According to this mid-sixteenth-century text, a person suffering from heat in the eyes should avoid sexual intercourse, the heat of the sun, and eating hot foods or condiments, such as "*chilimoli*," all of which increased heat in the body. The author further advised the sufferer to avoid looking at anything white and recommends various medicines that, once mixed with "woman's milk," should be dropped directly in the eyes.[45]

For diagnostic purposes, the hot/cold paradigm was easily linked to the larger processes playing themselves out in the Mesoamerican universe. Because the hot and cold properties of all beings and natural phenomena were detectable through the use of the senses, native healers had a tool through which they could interpret the mechanism of deities' actions. Depending on who caused an illness, a series of actions were set into motion, producing specific symptoms in the patient, which could then be read by the *titici*, or physician, and explained in terms of internal equilibrium and in changes of warmth or cold. Looking at Mesoamerican medicine through this schema helps us understand why, for example, Nahua healers differentiated between "hot" and "cold" fevers. Those that emanated from a celestial god would manifest themselves as "hot," while those that were derived from actions of the *tlaloques*, the earthly spirits of the *Tlaloque* deity group which lurked in streams and damp mountain ravines, were of a "cold" nature. The historical sources mention various kinds of wind, for example, such as the warm solar or celestial wind, *tona ehécatl*, or the cold aquatic wind, *ehécatl atl*, or the even more frigid airs, *mictlan ehécatl*, emanating from the dark underworld, all of which could shift the body into a state of disequilibrium.[46]

Again, we need to remind ourselves here how closely bodily equilibrium was tied to one's personal behavior. We have seen how sexual excess violated the Nahuas' ideal of moderation, but a whole host of other ideal forms of behavior were advocated as a way to minimize one's exposure to dangerous and chaotic forces. The *huehuetlatolli*, the "discourse of the elders" in the *Florentine Codex*, exhorts caution in all conduct of daily life such as speaking, dressing, eating and drinking. Clearly, these admonitions need to be viewed for what they are: ideals advocated by the ruling class, not accurate representations of how common Nahuas actually lived. Nonetheless, they provide the modern reader with a sense of the value system that helped to shape Postclassic Mesoamerican civilization. A person's form of speaking, for example, should be "moderately, middlingly," taking care "not to speak hurriedly, not to pant, nor to squeak, lest it be said of thee that thou art a groaner, a growler, a squeaker." One should not dress "vainly" or "fantastically," nor "place on thyself the gaudy cape, the gaudy clothing"; at the same time, one should not wear "rags, tatters, an old loosely-woven cape." Overeating and drunkenness both violated social moral codes, alhough the latter appears to have been a much weightier transgression: intoxication is frequently listed among the serious crimes—"pleasurable living," adultery, theft—mentioned by Sahagún's informants.[47] Indigenous drinking practices also shocked Spaniards who had their own ideals of moderation when it came to alcohol consumption, a topic that we look at in Chapter 4.

The Nahua elders cautioned against eating hastily or excessively. One should not "stir up the pieces [or] dig into the sauce bowl, the basket." So that one does not make a spectacle of oneself, one needs to eat calmly, quietly, not "gulp [food] like a dog."[48] Eating too quickly or too much was disorderly conduct that associated one with filth and with peoples and beasts of the periphery. One of the terms for glutton was *tlacazolli*, a composite of *tlacatl* "person" and the suffix–*zolli* "old and worn out" from the *tlazolli* complex, the words used to describe forms of pollution. The glutton was someone who aged before their time, reflecting the belief that the *tlazollii* in foods had a cumulative contaminating effect on the body.[49] The abhorrence that the Nahuas felt for such immoderation is clear in this very graphic description of a person who ingests the seeds of the *teopochotl* tree, which cause them to swell up like a glutton:

> That which is given as food, that which is given as drink then enlarges his body; it swells; it becomes in no place unblemished. Indeed, he becomes what is called a glutton—very fat, exceedingly fat, lazy, lumpy with flesh, round, an old clod of flesh with two eyes, heavy, very sluggish, a mass of leavened dough, big-headed; with ears like droplets, cylindrical eyelids, contracted eyes, fat cheeks, heavy cheeks, quivering cheeks, *tamal*- like nose, quivering nose, round nose; with thick lips, double chin, multiple chins; with flabby body, with hands like entrails; with filthy fingers, dirt-covered thighs, dirt-covered calves; with thick-soled feet . . . he becomes revolting; he just lies stretched out panting, breathing heavily. He has a great thirst, a great hunger; he eats three times, four times a day. All around he stores [food] for himself, and it is no little amount that he eats. He literally tramples upon the food.[50]

To overindulge in food or drink violated the ideal of equilibrium, as did too much physical comfort or idleness. That such ideals were strongly endorsed in pre-contact society sheds light on the ways in which native elders interpreted the high mortality rate in indigenous communities in the sixteenth century.

The natives who served as informants to the Spaniards compiling the *Relaciones Geográficas* repeatedly cited "the greater convenience (*el regalo*)" that life under Spanish rule brought to Mexico as the cause of so much death and disease, a life where people ate too often, ate too much meat and fat, drank too much alcohol, slept on soft beds, dressed too warmly, and had become lazy and idle.[51] To claim that Indians had a life of ease in a postconquest Mexico is of course an absurd assertion; what the elders were lamenting was the loss of a way of life grounded in ideals of balance and moderation.

Ostensibly, the Nahua medical model, which defined health as a state of equilibrium and charted vital changes in that equilibrium through a mapping of hot and cold qualities, appeared to share basic assumptions about the body with the medical model brought to Mexico in the early sixteenth century by Spaniards. Humoralism, a topic that we explore in depth in Chapter 4, also viewed health as a state of balance, although here the balance referred to the status of the four humors contained in the body; illness occurred when their natural balance was disturbed. The two systems had other similarities. Both were highly holistic, stressing the unity of the body, and the strong interaction between mental and physical processes. And both had similar notions about "ridding" the body of its disturbance, forcing the illness "out," usually through medications that purged. The Sahagún texts show that Nahua practitioners were as adept as their European counterparts when it came to purging, either via the stomach, intestines, or urinary track. Fevers were washed out in urine and expelled through the rectum or mouth.[52] Although superficial, such similarities facilitated the assimilation of Hippocratic ideas into Mexican culture. Ridding the body of its disorder through bleeding and purging was a widely used therapy throughout Mexico until modern medicine took hold in the early twentieth century, and even today lay people still refer to hot and cold qualities when discussing the cause of an illness. Yet, as the next chapter will show, the concepts Europeans had about their bodies could not have been more different from those of the pre-Conquest Nahuas.

NOTES

1. Louise M. Burkhart, *The Slippery Earth: Nahua-Christian Moral Dialogue in Sixteenth-Century Mexico* (Tucson: University of Arizona Press, 1989), p. 48; on Mesoamerican cosmology, see Miguel León Portilla, *Aztec Thought and Culture: A Study of the Ancient Nahuatl Mind*, trans. Jack Emory Davis (Norman: University of Oklahoma Press, 1963); David Carrasco, *Quetzalcoatl and the Irony of Empire: Myths*

and Prophecies in the Aztec Tradition (Chicago: University of Chicago Press, 1982); Alfredo López Austin, *The Human Body and Ideology: Concepts of the Ancient Nahuas*, trans. Thelma Ortiz de Montellano and Bernard Ortiz de Montellano, 2 vols. (Salt Lake City: University of Utah Press, 1988).

2. Burkhart, p. 48.

3. Bernard R. Ortiz de Montellano, *Aztec Medicine, Health, and Nutrition* (New Brunswick, NJ: Rutgers University Press, 1990), pp. 55–8; Burkhart, pp. 47–8.

4. Ortiz de Montellano, pp. 37–8.

5. Burkhart, p. 58.

6. López Austin, *The Human Body and Ideology*, Vol. I, p. 162.

7. Murray Last, "Non-Western Concepts of Disease," in CEHM, Vol. I, p. 643.

8. Ortiz de Montellano, pp. 61–2; Molina and *Relaciones Geográficas*, quoted in López Austin, *The Human Body and Ideology*, Vol. I, pp. 231–2.

9. Bernardino de Sahagún, *Florentine Codex. General History of the Things of New Spain*, ed. and trans. C. E. Dibble and A. J. O. Anderson, 12 books (Salt Lake City: University of Utah Press, 1950–69), Vol. XI, pp. 165, 171, 175, 188; *The Badianus Manuscript (Codex Barberini, Latin 241)*, ed. and trans. Emily Walcott Emmart (Baltimore: John Hopkins Press, 1940), p. 249.

10. Burkhart, pp. 49, 100.

11. Hernando Ruiz de Alarcón, *Treatise on the Heathen Superstitions That Today Live Among the Indians Native to This New Spain, 1629*, ed. and trans. J. Richards Andrews and Ross Hassig (Norman: University of Okalahoma Press, 1984), pp. 134–6; Burkhart, pp. 95–7; Ortiz de Montellano, p. 152.

12. Sahagún, *Florentine Codex*, II, p. 199.

13. Burkhart, pp. 117–24.

14. Sahagún, *Florentine Codex*, VI, p. 175.

15. López Austin, *The Human Body and Ideology*, Vol. I, p. 299; Sahagún, *Florentine Codex*, VI, pp. 142–3.

16. Ruiz de Alarcón, pp. 134–9.

17. Sahagún, *Florentine Codex*, IV, pp. 91 and VI, p. 257; Burkhart, pp. 110–11.

18. Carlos Viesca Treviño, *Medicina prehispánica*, p. 205.

19. Sahagún, *Florentine Codex*, XI, p. 191.

20. Burkhart, p. 99.

21. Sahagún, *Florentine Codex*, IV and V, p. 111.

22. López Austin, *The Human Body and Ideology*, Vol. I, pp. 220–21.

23. Ruiz de Alarcón, pp. 161–3.

24. Sahagún, *Florentine Codex*, VI, pp. 116–19.

25. Ortiz de Montellano, p. 153.

26. Sahagún, *Florentine Codex*, XI, pp. 183, 145, 170, and 174.

27. Sahagún, *Florentine Codex*, I, pp. 1–7.

28. Burkhart, p. 61.

29. Sahagún, *Florentine Codex*, III, pp. 11–12; IV and V, p. 171; I, p. 39; I, p. 31; III, 47.

30. Alarcón, p. 157; Viesca Treviño, *Medicina prehispánica*, pp. 80–1.

31. Burkhart, p. 59.

32. Sahagún, *Florentine Codex*, VI, p. 245.

33. Burkhart, p. 60.

34. Viesca Treviño, *Medicina prehispanica*, p. 82; Sahagún, *Florentine Codex*, I, p. 19.

35. Burkhart, p. 64; Sahagún, *Florentine Codex*, IV and V, pp. 151–80.

36. Sahagún, *Florentine Codex*, I. p. 39; Ortiz de Montellano, p. 163.

37. Sahagún, *Florentine Codex*, I, pp. 23–7 and VI, pp. 29–34.

38. Burkhart, pp. 181–3.

39. Sahagún, *Florentine Codex*, IV and V, p. 101; Ortiz de Montellano, pp. 140–1; Viesca Teviño, *Medicina prehispanica*, pp. 88–94.

40. Jacques Soustelle, "Apuntes sobre la psicología y el sistema de valores en México antes de la conquista," in *Estudios antropológocps publicados en homenaje al Doctor Manuel Gamio* (México: Universidad Nacional Autónoma de México, 1950).

41. Sahagún, *Florentine Codex*, VI, p. 110.

42. Burkhart, pp. 130–4.

43. López Austin, *The Human Body and Ideology*, pp. 260–1.

44. Sahagún, *Florentine Codex*, XI, pp. 146, 153, 157, 166.

45. *The Badianus Manuscript*, pp. 218, 252, 260, 289.

46. Viesca Treviño, *Medicina prehispanica*, pp. 104–5.

47. Sahagún, *Florentine Codex*, VI, pp. 87–139, quotes on pp. 122–3; Burkhart, p. 160.

48. Sahagún, *Florentine Codex*, VI, p. 124.

49. Burkhart, p. 160.

50. Sahagún, *Florentine Codex*, XI, pp. 215–16.

51. PNE, pp. 224, 245–6; RG, Vol. VI, p. 88.

52. Sahagún, *Florentine Codex*, XI, pp. 142, 143, 149, 153, 159, and 166.

4. MANAGING THE HUMORS

In July 1757, the Condesa de Miravalle noted in a letter to her son-in-law that she had been so busy attending to sick family members that she had not even had time to purge herself. An author of one of the *Relaciones Geográficas* from the sixteenth century remarked that the Indians of Cuicatlan were usually healthy, although they sometimes got fevers from eating too much fruit. And in his account of their journey through Mexico in the 1580s, Antonio de Ciudad Real described the experience Fray Alonoso Ponce had when he fell deathly ill with *dolor de ijada*. According to the chronicler, the cause of the illness was self-evident: it came from "the [rain] water that fell on him, and the excessive cold he experienced from Xalapa to Quechúlac, such that,—all of this entered his side [*ijada*] and took root there, so that in order to cure him, many *beneificios* were necessary . . ."[1]

Each of these anecdotes is revealing. Collectively they confirm that ordinary people—that is, those outside the circle of medically trained professionals—had well-formed ideas about what constituted a threat to health. Examined more closely, they display some of those notions being applied in daily life. To maintain the body's humoral balance, a periodic purging or bleeding was viewed as an especially beneficial prophylaxis; food, with its elaborate qualities—hot and cold, wet and dry—directly influenced the inner workings of the body, hence its heavy medicinal use as well; and exposure to all sorts of environmental hazards—excessive heat, cold, or humidity, sudden temperature changes, bad air, and putrid vapors—produced dangerous physiological changes.

Behind these lay notions about illness were particular ideas about the nature of disease and the inner workings of the human body. Here we explore these ideas through the prism of European medicine, a body of thought imported into Mexico during the very first years of the viceroyalty and the only legally sanctioned medical model throughout the three hundred years of colonial rule. Early modern medicine was based largely on humoralism, a set of anatomical and physical ideas inherited from ancient Greek medicine. Although these theories were quite elaborate and not fully accessible to many outside a small circle of educated professionals and laypeople, the basic notions about the human body that underlay them were widely accepted in the general population. Apart from divine or supernatural causes, the most common threat to human health lay in the environment and in one's own daily lifestyle. Consequently, a large part of early modern medicine was as concerned with preventive health care as it was with the treatment of disease. Ideally, the practitioner sought to maintain a patient's health by regulating his or her environmental conditions, diet, exercise, rest, and psychological well-being. Our point of entry here will be to delve into that body of advice lore, proffered by contemporary experts, which emerged around the classical rules of hygiene, or what today we would call preventive medicine. When viewed with other colonial sources—personal letters, chronicles, travelers' accounts—this point of intersection between medical theory and daily life, which was the area of academic medicine that was most accessible to laypeople, contains invaluable clues about an important part of everyday life in colonial Mexico, namely, how people thought about and managed their health. It also provides another angle from which to view Europeans making sense of the new climates, foods, and peoples of their colonial possessions.

EUROPEAN ORIGINS: HUMORALISM

Humoralism first emerged in the fifth century BC in the Greek communities of Ionia (Asia Minor) and the Greek mainland, and for more than two millennia it formed the basis of the Western medical tradition. Although its theories were continually being revised by later scholars, its main features remained recognizable up to the birth of modern medicine in the nineteenth century. Its most basic premise was that a person's health was the result of a natural balance of the four main bodily fluids, or humors, and that illness resulted from a disturbance in that balance. The early Hippocratic texts on medicine depicted the body in constant flux making health precarious as it was continually exposed to the harmful influences from one's diet, lifestyle, and the environment. Thus, a diagnosis of a particular illness was a complicated matter, as so many factors, both inside and outside the body, might be involved. Yet if the right balance of humors could be found, health could be restored and, with a good deal of prophylaxis, be maintained as well. Humoralism was a holistic medical system: it stressed the unity of the individual, the connection between mental and physical processes. It also was both highly individualist—in that each individual had their own natural humoral composition, or temperament—and universal, because the variation of diseases was not unlimited and the same pattern of illness could afflict many individuals.[2]

One of the most important developments of classical Greek thinking was its promotion of natural explanations for the phenomena of the world. In the field of medicine, this led to the search for natural explanations of disease, a major departure from medical systems that saw illness originating from supernatural entities, either as divine punishment or the manipulations of people with special powers. In the Hippocratic text *On the Sacred Disease*, the author explicitly ridiculed the idea that epilepsy was caused by divine forces and in fact none of the works of the Hippocratic Corpus, the earliest writings on humoralism, contain any mention of disease being caused or cured by the gods. These early writings were later synthesized in the second century AD by Galen of Pergamum (now Bergama, Turkey), who united clinical Hippocratic medicine into a theoretical framework. Galen produced and promoted a vast opus of some 350 works ranging on such topics as bloodletting, the pulse, and the soul. Translations of the Galenic and Hippocratic texts into Arabic in the ninth century spread humoralism throughout Muslim lands and during the Middle Ages these same texts were introduced into the Latin West, forming the basis of learned medicine for the next millennium. The Galenic system linked the four elements and their qualities—fire (warm), water (cold), earth (dry), wind (moist)—with the four humors in the body: bile (warm-dry), phlegm (cold-moist), black bile (cold-dry), and blood (warm-moist). The natural mixture of these humors determined an individual's temperament, most people having one or a pair of humors in predominance, which, in turn, determined psychological as well as physical disposition. A vestige of this belief survives today in the English adjectives sanguine, phlegmatic, choleric, and melancholy to describe personality traits.[3] That medical theories and therapies would have centered on bodily fluids is understandable. The word "humor" comes from the Greek word for fluid or juice. Because all living things have some form of fluid—sap in plants, blood in animals—assigning them a vital part in the physical process of life made perfect sense to people in ancient times who based their understanding of the world solely on its observable phenomena.[4]

A large part of classical and early modern medical writing was concerned with what today we would regard as preventive medicine, or what the Greeks called "hygiene" or "regimen." Today, hygiene's association with health is mostly limited to ideas of cleanliness; since the nineteenth century, the germ theory of disease—the idea that microorganisms can cause illness—has made us aware of the role cleanliness plays in the maintenance of health. The classical view of hygiene, however, was not necessarily concerned with keeping clean but with personal lifestyle and one's relationship to the environment. Climate and geographical location, food and drink, patterns of sleeping and waking, the retentions and evacuations of the body, motion and rest, and one's emotional state were all taken into account when explaining and curing sickness. Sometime after Galen, these were often referred to as the six "nonnaturals," a term with mysterious origins and somewhat confusing connotations because they were indeed natural processes of the body. In his *Ars Medica*, Galen explained why hygiene was so important for one's health:

> Of necessity we are immersed in the surrounding air, and we eat, drink, wake and sleep. We are not necessarily thrust against swords or beasts. Hence in the first category of causes but not in the second there is an art devoted to the protection of the body. Now that these matters have been set forth, we shall find in each of these items which necessarily alter the body, its own kind of healthful causes. One comes from contact with the surrounding air, another from movement and rest of the whole body or its parts, a third from sleep and waking, a fourth from things taken into the body, a fifth from those that are excreted and returned, a sixth from affections of the mind.[5]

The six nonnaturals were not viewed solely as prophylaxis but as a framework on which to structure therapies as well. The intake of medicine figured into the category of food and drink, bleeding and purgatives were an important element of bodily evacuations, and much attention was given to the type of environment or air best suited for curing ailments. A patient's emotional state was not to be neglected either; passing time in the countryside with pleasant company might prove more effective than the most potent elixir.[6]

The theory of humors was further strengthened, and complicated, by coordinating them to the time of year and to the stage of one's life. Thus, a particular humor predominated during each season and at different ages of a particular individual. Blood, for example, was more abundant in young children and in everyone during the spring, resulting in more diseases caused by a *plethora* of blood, such as spring fever or bloody noses. In summertime, and during youth, the hotter and drier yellow bile predominated; black bile in the fall and throughout adulthood; and phlegm, being cold and wet, increased in winter and in old age. Linking the four qualities with observable phenomena not only boosted the explanatory force of the medical model; it also provided the doctor with some foundational information by knowing in advance just what humor was likely to be predominant and which were likely to be deficient. Of course, this added to the complexity of diagnosis because one's stage in life did not necessarily correspond to the season and each person had their own humoral composition.[7]

It is not difficult to see why humoralism became so dominant in Europe and in the Islamic world. Its ability to explain almost anything made it both credible and unfalsifiable, provided one accepted its premises, which according to Galen were "common notions," or "what everyone knew." Moreover, its errors could easily be ascribed to the practitioner or patient, not to the system itself. Perhaps its real strength was that it offered a basis for treatment, and, even more important in an age before effective medicine, for prophylaxis, that to a large extent corresponded to what the patient might observe. Many illnesses do tend to be more common at certain times of the year, attack certain age groups and not others, and seem to get better after treatment.[8] In other words, because of its inclusiveness, flexibility, and accessibility the system worked well for physician and patient alike, which helps to explain its long dominance in Western culture.

Above all, to the physician it offered the apparent certitude of an effective system of practice. Its very antiquity, even to Galen, helped to confirm its authority. Its regularity provided a method for controlling health and disease, by both intervention and prophylaxis, while at the same time its emphasis on the individuality of each patient and ultimately of each condition gave ample opportunity for practitioners to display their skills and their learning in understanding that individuality and in prescribing accordingly. Yet, as a system, it was sufficiently simple for many patients to grasp, and even thereby to treat themselves, and hence to join with their physician in a combined attack on disease. The very accessibility of humoralism may well have helped to establish the credentials of those who put its theories into practice at the bedside, and has given the patient added confidence in what was being done, simply through being able to follow what was being said or prescribed.[9]

Thus, as a framework for conceptualizing how the body worked, humoralism's great advantage lay in its accessibility to the layman. Like other aspects of their European culture—and that part of a culture concerned with the constraints of life and death, health and disease, surely is one of its most significant—the humoral medical model was fundamental to a Spanish understanding of the natural world. During the early years of New Spain's existence, it was dominant only where Spanish settlement occurred. Because they rejected indigenous medical practices, Spaniards set about importing their own medical institutions, personnel, and knowledge from the mother country. But as Spanish and, later, Europeanized mestizo communities, grew, so did humoral medicine. Although other medical approaches—indigenous medicine, Christian faith healing, rituals based on magic—robustly functioned alongside it, and, indeed, were incorporated into its methods, humoralism eventually became the dominant way of understanding the body in nonreligious terms by the late colonial years.

HAZARDOUS ENVIRONMENTS AND RISKY BEHAVIOR

Juan de Esteyneffer begins his eighteenth-century medical guide, *Florilegio medicinal de todas las enfermedades,* with some general information about why people become ill. Disease causes fall into two large categories, he writes: the first group consists of "intrinsic" or interior causes, that is, they come from the humors themselves, which sometimes "make sick the inside of the body and all its parts"; the second type, the "extrinsic" or external causes, are much more common:

> These are called so because they are offered outside the human body, by which they alter and vary its maladies, [they are] the air, food and drink, sleep and awakeness, movement or exercise and rest, evacuations and retentions, passions of the mind [*los accidentes o pasiones del ánimo*]. All are necessary and all affect the body. Those maintained in a measured and proportioned manner conserve the body's health, and those lacking or exceeding in proportion cause disease. And these are the most ordinary causes outside of others that sometimes appear.[10]

Esteyneffer's medical ideas, which were representative of learned medicine in the Americas and Europe in the last half of the seventeenth century, were still solidly based on a Greek medicine as it was first theorized in the Hippocratic Corpus, and later by Galen and Arabian authors. The art of hygiene, used here in its classical sense, formed the foundation for this medicine. As a holistic approach to health, it was primarily concerned with how one's body was affected by the environment and one's own lifestyle, and each of the six nonnaturals were separate factors around which preventative and therapeutic strategies were organized. As ideas about what caused disease began to change in the nineteenth century, and the nonnaturals became secondary, medicine lost it holistic quality. By the time scientists discovered that bacteria and viruses were the primary causes of infectious disease in the twentieth century, the concept of hygiene had similarly lost its holistic perspective, making dirt and hidden germs the motives behind modern hygienic practices. Social and cultural changes also influenced this evolution. In the eighteenth century, the elaboration of manners in the upper classes began to change standards of cleanliness, notions that filtered down to the middle classes in the following century. And although Christianity had always imposed moral and even ascetic overtones onto notions of hygiene (the sins of gluttony and drunkenness!), the shift to an emphasis on cleanliness cemented its association with moral worth in the modern collective mind. Not all classical conceptions of hygiene have been lost, however. Lifestyle still forms a part of medicine, and increasingly so because what tends to kill us now are chronic ailments, many of which are associated with how we live. These are links to an older concept of hygiene, which has now lost its name.[11]

People's ideas about the ages and stages of life were firmly linked to concepts about personal hygiene. The rules for good hygiene reflected the Hippocratic notion that different regimens and measures had to be appropriate to the age of the individual. The idea of the ages of man is, of course, an old one, with roots reaching far back into literature, religion, and medical theory. The Galenic view was that an individual's life span was fixed by nature; thus, the goal of proper hygiene was to reach the allotted number of years. During the Middle Ages and Renaissance, however, a more active and malleable view of nature slowly evolved in which the human life span could be prolonged with the right regimen. Much of the medical advice from this period advocated special remedies, diets, exercise, and bathing regimes to extend natural lifetimes.[12]

Christobal Méndez, a sixteenth-century Spanish physician who wrote one of the earliest books promoting the virtues of exercise in Europe, included two chapters on the stages of life. "Everyone knows there are six ages," he writes, and "everybody should remember them to preserve his health and to know in what age he is included." The early years of life were classified similarly to our own modern notions of childhood: the period of infancy consisted of the first three years, when children should be rocked in their cradles "with sweet and pleasant singing"; and, from three to fourteen years, the age of childhood, "because up till then, man preserves his innocence." Méndez's advice for parents includes keeping children (almost all of his advice applies only to boys and men, as females were excluded from vigorous activity) away from games that were played for profit, like bowling or card games, because they are likely to "pick up bad attitudes which are dangerous." Also, if children are too active after eating, "they may suffer that unhappy disease, stone in the bladder." The third stage of life, adolescence, which continues to twenty-five years, is when people have their best health, "the period when we suffer least from work." The fourth stage, through age forty or forty-five, "when men are in complete strength and vigor" is youth; the appropriate form and amount of exercise is very important at this time of life, writes Méndez, because "if we do not do what is necessary to consume and expend [the superfluities], diseases attack that give trouble in old age like torments in the side and kidneys, gout, and the disease of stones." The last two stages, old age—up to seventy years—and the remaining years of very old age or "decrepitude," are the periods in life in which people "have very weak natural heat [and] the superfluities increase." Gentle movement and temperance in everything is the rule for old people. Proper exercise includes riding a mule, slow walking, and for very old men, being rocked "very gently in cradles because as they return to the age of children we have to give them the same kind of exercise."[13]

The human life span, then, could be viewed as a gradual process by which the body slowly lost its natural heat and, according to Juan de Cárdenas, the humidity that fueled it.

> . . . natural death . . . is when a man without any type of illness, but only from pure old age, dies for lack of any trace of the natural heat that has sustained him, and this he loses because he has used up that sustaining humidity, in which this natural heat is conserved.[14]

Life often was compared to a lamp or candle that would naturally extinguish itself when its fuel had been used up. "The light lasts as long as the natural heat and humidity of the oil does . . . as soon as any one of these qualities are lacking, it dies and goes out, and so is the life of man." One started out in life with plenty of heat; children and adolescents were naturally "hot" (even more so if their individual complexions were dominated by one of the hot humors), thus foods that warmed the body were only to be eaten with precaution. This age group, too, needed more circulating air in their sleeping rooms than other age groups so that it will "temper the fire and heat of their boiling humors." The progressive loss of this body heat was visible in the gray hair older people acquired. When heat left the body, the cold and wet humor phlegm took its place, and since "its own natural color is white, the force of its excretions . . . turned the hair white, because the hair is nothing but some humors and excretions which result from the humors of our bodies."[15] One's personal regimen, then, was intimately tied to one's stage of life as well as to everyday health maintenance.

INVASIVE AIRS

From the moment that humans began to find explanations for their illnesses in the natural elements of their own world, rather than in divine causation, the human milieu has been viewed as a prominent provoker of disease. Exposure to cold or hot winds, the sun's harsh rays, cold rain, proximity to lakes and marshes, and such urban features as cemeteries, public latrines, and garbage dumps were all believed to directly influence the inner workings of the body. In a myriad of ways, the environment posed a major health hazard. In the early years of the twenty-first century, the idea that external conditions play a part in the occurrence of disease is not an alien concept to us. The degenerative and chronic diseases that are the prime causes of morbidity and mortality in Western societies today are now frequently linked with changes in the environment. Modern studies confirm that sustained exposure to chemical and radioactive materials can cause some cancers, and our polluted air creates serious respiratory problems in many people. Although the particular aspects of the environment that are singled out as being unhealthy may have changed over the centuries, the linking of disease to conditions in the world that surrounds us is therefore not a new phenomenon.

For practitioners of Galenic medicine, illness was simply an imbalance in the humors of the body; not so simple, however, was knowing what upset this balance in the first place. Any variation or excess in personal regimen was always suspect, a topic we turn to below, but beyond this, were the elements of the environment that might trigger an episode of illness. It was common knowledge that climate produced physiological changes; everyone knew, for example, that cold and damp weather led to colds and excessive heat to fevers. Certain endemic diseases seemed to be connected with certain geographical locations and weather patterns. And epidemics, which inexplicably inflicted the same symptoms on many people at the same time, frequently were blamed on bad or corrupted air.

One of the first texts in the Hippocratic Corpus to address the connection between the environment and health, *Airs, Waters, Places*, written sometime in fifth century BC, was designed to enable the practitioner to anticipate what diseases he was likely to observe in a new, unfamiliar town. According to this foundational text, both the cold north wind and south hot wind were best avoided for the threat of disease they contained. Topographical features such as altitude, exposure to winds, nearness to rivers, lakes, or forests also were critical factors when choosing a place to live or a travel route, as was the quality of water. The most dangerous waters were ones that were stagnant, such as those found in marshlands, or those emanating from a ground source, while the best waters came from high places. And rainwater, although praised as light, sweet, and clear, could quickly turn foul.[16]

Classical ideas on the connections between the environment and health show up often in colonial Mexican sources. The *Relaciones Geográficas*, the detailed questionnaire that circulated throughout New Spain between the years

1578 and 1585, contains numerous examples of Spanish preoccupation with the connections between geography, climate, and disease. Among the many questions generated in this ambitious project was one that asked if a town or site was healthy or not. The answers reveal a lot about lay perceptions of disease causation. The *Relación de Chinantla*, for example, says that "[this place] is hot, humid, and sick: it rains eight months of the year; for three months big, cold north winds blow, which cause the Indians to get sick with coughs and colds, and sometimes they get *dolor de costado*. The wind rules this province."[17] Heat and dampness were dangerous to health, as was cold wind, but warmth and dryness were good: the town of Taxco "was more healthy than its surroundings, even though it is naturally hot, because . . . the high location makes it airy and from this it is moderately hot and dry."[18] But too much dampness, not only from rain, but in the form of fog, mists, or evening dew as well could make one vulnerable to illness. "The *Villa de Tepuztlan*, is an unhealthy place because it is in a valley between some mountains . . . where, as there flows much water, there is an unusual amount of humidity and fog, which causes a heavy evening mist (*serenos*) . . ."[19] The Indian *pueblo* of Chimalhuacan is unhealthy because of "the great quantity of humidity it has and from the vapor of the lagoon that is near it, and for the many sources of water and springs there are here . . ."[20]

Personal accounts of illness also testify to the unshakable conviction people had about the role weather played in their health. Exposure to extremes of temperature, especially to coldness when it was accompanied by wetness almost always prophesied serious illness. A letter writer in the sixteenth century recounts for relatives back home the frightening accident he had while traveling near Puebla on horseback in December of 1559 and the resulting "*año de enfermedad*" that followed.

> . . . a horse fell with me into the river, and it was my misfortune that this happened during freezing weather . . . the way out was a wet and frozen slope of a ravine, made into a hard icicle . . . the horse slipped on all four legs and fell onto his back with me in the water, and, God being served, I was not caught underneath, and from this fall I did not have one thread of dry clothing left. . . . I wiped myself off as I had no way to obtain dry clothes, and all that cold entered my gut [*en las tripas*], so that I suffered from the pain of it until the month of April, and as my pain was getting better with the hot weather, all my limbs were becoming crippled, so much so that I could not even bring a jug of water to my mouth. . . . I had to put myself under care in August and was nine days "in sweats" [*en sudores*], and first I spent my money on stupid doctors, and after that, God being served, I found a doctor who in twenty days cured me.[21]

In another letter written by a barber-surgeon in service to a local convent, we see that going out at night can lead to all sorts of health problems. "Of my health," he writes, "I have been at times very badly indisposed, and it is because of the work I do at the convent of the friars, who get up at one or two o'clock in the morning, and the evening mist [*sereno*] in this land is so bad, it has damaged me horribly, and in truth has reduced the days of my life . . ."[22]

Just how did humidity work with inclement temperatures to threaten the body? The letters' authors do not explain this, nor presumably did laypeople sense the need to conceptualize this process in a formal manner. It was generally understood that a wet chill could cause a disequilibrium of the humors somewhere in body; this knowledge was simply what everyone knew, a commonsense notion. Underlying this conception, however, was a very specific image: the penetrable body whose skin was seen as porous, creating countless openings through which damaging substances could easily slip in. The combination of heat and water was viewed as especially dangerous because hot temperatures opened up the pores, allowing the damaging effects of water to enter the body and upset the equilibrium of the humors. In the *Relación de Zapotitlán*, the author writes that the Indians of "these towns" often get *pasmo*, a "dangerous disease" that comes because "there are torrential downpours here and, as the land is hot, [this causes] the pores to open, and if a remedy is not applied right away, fever comes, and later the *pasmo*."[23] The same kind of disease causes are cited by Bernardo de Vargas Machuca, a professional soldier who spent more than twenty years in military campaigns in the New World. In his book, *Milicia y descripción de Las Indias*, which might be described as a conquistador's handbook, Vargas Machuca devotes a special chapter to the treatment of wounds and illness. Colds are the most common ailments in the military, he writes, because "these lands are so hot and the soldier is always marching on foot and sweating . . . his body becomes hot and open [*abierta las carnes*], then he becomes sick. The same happens when passing rivers or in downpours, which are never lacking."[24] This permeability of the skin proved to be a constant source of anxiety for European inhabitants in the New World. The climate—with its extremes of heat, moisture, and cold—opened up the body's surface to a whole host of elements that threatened to upset the delicate balance of humors.

The fog and mist that forms during the night were viewed by Spaniards as an especially perilous element of the environment. Juan de Cárdenas devotes a chapter of *Primera parte de los problemas y secretos de la Indias* to the question of: "Why is the night mist [*sereno*] in the Indies so much more harmful than in other places?" He cites two reasons: one, because the sereno is so plentiful in the Indies; and second, because the bodies "of those of us that live [here] are very abundant in humidity, which notably increases and doubles with the sereno." Cárdenas wants, first of all, to edify his readers on the general subject of how cold moisture affects the body, "because a thousand times we hear about the damage and effects it causes us, and hardly is there a disease for which we do not make it the inventor."[25] Because most people are confused about what constitutes sereno and what its qualities are, Cárdenas provides a definition:

> . . . sereno is nothing more than that subtle and delicate vapor, that, having risen during the day with the warmth of the sun, becomes condensed with the cold of the night. The properties and natural qualities of this vapor, or sereno, are coldness and humidity which have great subtlety and penetration. . . . We can infer thus, that the more humidity there is in the land, as there is strength in the sun to raise this vapor, there will be a greater quantity of vapor . . . [26]

The Indies, Cárdenas writes elsewhere in the book, has an abundance of humidity, because of its many bodies of water in the form of rivers, marshes, and lagoons. Furthermore, there "is always heat in great quantity."[27] This combination of copious sunshine and abundant water made it a natural place for heavy night mist.

Cárdenas's other explanation for why sereno is so dangerous in the New World is that people of European descent who live there seem to acquire a great deal of humidity or phlegm in their bodies. This comes from simply being in a humid environment, but also from faulty hygiene: ". . . from the little exercise they do, from too much food and drink, and even from too many carnal acts that many here engage in." Consequently, this excess humidity "swells the body with excrements, which, little by little, and without illness, strangles its natural heat and shortens life."[28] Climate—in this case, the excessive humidity—combines with lifestyle to play an important role in everyday health. In classic humoral theory, Cárdenas reasons that any shift toward an excess or deficiency in one of the body's humors will set off a *destemplanza,* or an imbalance in the system: "as experience shows us, when a body undergoes a *destemplanza,* it will receive more damage when more similar things are applied to that *destemplanza,* for example, if a man is imbalanced with too much cold, it is clear that the more cold things we apply to him, the more impaired he will become."[29] In the case of sereno, then, its abundance in the atmosphere combines with the excess of phlegm in European bodies to threaten health.

Hot climates also generated a great deal of concern about one's vulnerability to disease. Coming from subtropical zones with more temperate climates, Spaniards were unaccustomed to the awesome heat and humidity of the tropical regions of Mexico. For the most part, these areas were viewed as extremely unhealthy, but not always. Antonio de Ciudad Real's impression of Yucatan's climate is generally a favorable one, although the humidity, as always, is problematic. It is, he writes, "extremely hot, but very healthy, especially for old people, because of the good air and provisions it has. It is very humid, and because of this, not healthy for legs but good for heads." It also rates more favorably because, as it lacks rivers, it has fewer mosquitoes than other areas the traveling friars had visited.[30]

In general, however, Spaniards viewed the tropical coasts of Mexico as unhealthy places in which to live and through which to travel. The surgeon Pedro Arias de Benavides warns those traveling to the New World that they should "leave the ports as soon as possible and go to the interior because there the land is healthy and even if they get sick it is not of great consequence, which is quite the contrary in the sea ports for the great amount of heat there is in them."[31] The archetype of all sickly locations, of course, was Vera Cruz, a place that generated a plethora of negative commentary throughout the three centuries of Spanish rule, and was often referred to as *la tumba de los españoles* because of its association with the *vómito prieto*, or yellow fever. The author of the *Relación de la ciudad de Veracruz* gives an extensive account of why the site is so unhealthy:

> . . . [Vera Cruz] is naturally unhealthy, for many and strong reasons . . . besides being situated in a low place, and being naturally humid, and being sheltered from the healthful winds, and open to the unhealthful ones, it is also very hot here for most of the year . . .

The heat—or, more precisely, the sun—causes several things to happen that makes this particular location so insalubrious. The sun's rays are so "strong and direct" and the resulting landscape of "sand dunes and hills of dead sand, without a tree or living plant," are so desolate that the sun strikes and "wounds with a vehemence." This, in turn, causes:

> . . . many exhalations and hot vapors to rise, which seize and burn the atmosphere in this infamous region . . . [and] with this excessive heat, the blood boils and *cólera* begins to grow, which causes [in the body] a surplus of heat, [intensified by] the humidity and rains, that in this land are incessant during the summer and part of the fall . . . [all this] generates many dangerous diseases caused by the corruption of the humors . . .

Extremely hot weather threatens the body by raising its internal temperature to a dangerous level. In addition, the unhealthy winds magnify the body's compromised state: "not only do they enfeeble and weaken the natural forces, but they also unleash the humors and corrupt them, especially when, together with the rain and heat of summer, they begin to blow." The author of this *relación* further cites the sudden shifts in temperature that tend to occur in coastal climates such as Vera Cruz's, noting that "the weather changes that commonly happen here alter bodies notably."[32] Nearly two hundred years later, the same kinds of observations were being made on the diseased state of this city. The Capuchine friar, Francisco de Ajofrín, who disembarked there in 1763, remarked that: "all the people who live here, even the young people, are of pallid complexion, and are in such a broken state of health [*tan quebrados*], as if they were convalescing from a grave illness, and the cause is the continual transpiration and sweating from the excessive heat, [which is] seen also in their actions and even in they way they speak . . ."[33] High temperatures, humidity, the sun, and harmful winds all combined to make Vera Cruz a pestilential place.

These classical notions about health and the environment were part of the framework Europeans used to make sense of foreign lands and different climates. Basic to Galenic conceptions of the body was the idea that an individual's temperament, or *complexión*, was partly determined by the environment, especially the climate of one's birthplace. A move to a different land exposed one to a new climate that might not be compatible with one's natural temperament thus putting the body at risk. Europeans struggling to adapt to new environments were especially vulnerable to heat and humidity which tended to "weaken" their constitutions. A period of "seasoning," or gradual adaptation, not only to climate but also to new foods and drinks as well, could restore strength to a compromised constitution.[34]

In the last half of the eighteenth century, educated commentators' observations on the connections between climate and disease became decidedly more "scientific." In his popular *Mercurio volante, con noticias importantes y curiosas sobre física y medicina*, José Ignacio Bartolache described with excitement the new instruments used for charting weather patterns, the thermometer and barometer. Shortly thereafter, a series of articles written in the spring of 1784 in *La Gaceta de México* explained for readers how they aid in "observing the condition of the air that surrounds us." The weather conditions of several months were exhaustingly described with great precision, but the connections between temperature, humidity, and health remained essentially the same as they were in the sixteenth century. The unusual amount of humidity during the fall of 1783 caused a rise in *dolor de costado, insultos, pulmonías*; a sudden drop in temperature in February caused these ailments to increase even more, along with "fluxes of the eyes" and fever in children.[35] The development of instruments for measuring such things as rainfall, temperature, and wind velocity stimulated further efforts to quantify climatic conditions. Yet, rather than challenge centuries-old notions about disease causation and the environment, the new instrument-based observations tended to reinforce them.[36]

MIASMA

Colonials, then, had to be mindful of the climate and its potentially harmful affects on their health. But sudden temperature shifts and penetrating moisture were not the only dangers the environment held; everyone knew that it possessed a much more horrifying threat, jeopardizing not just isolated individuals, but large sections of the population as well. For concealed in the surrounding atmosphere was the threat of pestilence. Today, our understanding of epidemic disease is based on concepts of bacteriology and virology. Even most lay people know that infectious disease is caused by microorganisms that invade the body and then is spread either by person-to-person or person-vector-person transmission chains. In this biomedical model, the environment plays a minor role. Up to the nineteenth century, however, people conceptualized epidemics in a fundamentally different way. As one medical historian put it: "Far from regarding epidemic diseases as distinct in origin from environmental maladies, [people] commonly viewed them as a special case—by far the most serious—of disease induced by the environment."[37] In this view, pestilence came from the air itself.

According to a report put out by the Protomedicato in 1696, the noxious air in Mexico City had several sources: the vapors or exhalations coming from the muddy shores of lakes and lagoons, which, with the heat of the sun, become foul smelling and poisonous; a cold winter followed by extreme heat in the summer, which causes the fish and other aquatic animal life to rot and corrupt the air with their odor; shallowly dug gravesites; an accumulation of human and animal fecal material in parts of the capital; the large amount of garbage found in the city; and the wasteful practice of slaughterhouses which killed more animals than needed, leaving the extra carcasses to rot in the streets.[38]

The particular causes singled out by the Protomedicato were all based on centuries-old conceptions of miasma, or the idea that "corrupted" air itself was a significant cause of disease. In their attempt to explain epidemics naturalistically, the Hippocratic authors cited the air as a cause of illness and its tainting by miasma as the reason why so many people could be struck with the same set of symptoms at the same time. In early Greek writings, miasma was associated with notions of staining or tainting, and ideas of pollution. The exact way in which miasma transmitted disease was not explicitly clear, but the process was often reflected in analogies and metaphors that mirrored the workings of the natural world. Some of the examples offered to explain what happened to air to make it pathological were the rotting of fruit, in which decay spread from one part of the fruit to another, or the processes of dyeing cloth or fermentation in wine-making.[39] How were miasmatic places identified? Before the age of chemical analysis of air, water, and soil, the health hazards of the environment had to be judged by an individual's senses. The common feature that seemed to link them was foul odor, and, for this reason, such malodorous sites as marshes, slaughterhouses, tanneries, cesspools, cemeteries, and refuse dumps were singled out as sources of corrupted air.

In colonial Mexico, the repeated cycles of epidemic disease understandably created anxiety and panic in the population, especially for those living in urban settings. And although colonial authorities in the sixteenth and seventeenth centuries were preoccupied with containing the sources of tainted air, it was not until the eighteenth century, during the reign of the reform-minded Bourbons, that these efforts became conceptualized as a concern for public health as a whole. This period coincided with a general renewed interest in the West of Hippocratic concepts linking the environment with health, although now the model of hygiene was shifting from an emphasis on the individual to one based on the collective.[40] The obvious remedy for stagnant and corrupted air was to somehow get it circulating. Many ideas were offered, ranging from the practical to the ridiculous. In 1763, the viceroy, the Marqués de Cruillas, mentioned in an *informe* on yellow fever that it was necessary "to clear away the mountains at a distance of one league from populations so that the air might circulate . . ." The uninhibited flow of air was also a concern of city planners. One observer in the eighteenth century noted that streets should be laid out long and wide, without "torturous recesses," so that when the wind blows "it will sweep away the fog and clean the atmosphere of any harmful humidity." The Protomedicato offered other pragmatic suggestions: "the streets and ditches should be clean . . . that under no circumstances should dead bodies be left in the commercial district, nor on street corners; that graves should be dug deeply; that of the Indians coming into the city, the sick ones should be kept at the hospital, and the healthy ones returned to their pueblos."[41] The Protomedicato's declarations also demonstrate the widespread belief that the air was fouled not only from substances above ground but from below it as well. The preoccupation with burying the dead in deeply dug graves sprang from the fear that as dead bodies decayed, they released corrupting vapors into the air. The same dangers materialized with earthquakes, which left crevices in the ground, or for laborers when they descended to work in mines, and even by cultivation, which released trapped vapors hidden in the soil. These commonly accepted notions engendered a preoccupation with fissures, faults, and the boundaries of any dangerous terrain, where noxious vapors might ascend into the atmosphere and endanger human bodies.[42]

If the environment played such a large role in the cause and spread of disease, it would seem there was little that people could do to protect themselves. Yet, there is nothing in the historical record to show that people were passive or fatalistic about the threat of disease coming from their surroundings. The familiar dictum of 'flee quickly and far' was advice people undoubtedly followed when they could, but not everyone could flee; knowing how to insulate themselves from pestilence at home was therefore crucial. Home-care manuals and newspapers were full of prophylactic advice. In an article on the smallpox epidemic that struck Mexico in 1779, José Ignacio Bartolache tells readers that a bit of fine vinegar applied to the mouth and nose may offer protection from the current pestilence. Esteyneffer advises readers to eat rue leaves every morning along with bread, fresh butter and honey, or a bit of a paste made from figs and nuts as a prophylactic against pestilence. He also mentions that "some use with good effect the drinking of one's own urine . . . for protection in contagious times." And if controlling the macro-environment was impossible, at least people could attend to their own micro-environments. Well-ventilated rooms, with fresh air flowing freely, were of paramount importance as was the use of aromatic substances to purify the air. One health manual recommended "spraying the sleeping chamber many times with rosewater and vinegar, and put[ting] green herbs in the room, as well as things like willow branches, vine leaves, cypress, scape, or green reeds." Another noted the benefit of always carrying a piece of juniper root on one's person, "the frequent smelling of which is good protection against the *peste*." Collectively, too, in villages and cities alike, people tried to cleanse the air with bonfires or by shooting off canons.[43]

Such tactics confirm that colonial Mexicans viewed the ungovernable environment as a major source of illness, even though they could at least take some personal action to protect themselves from its dangers. But contemporary etiology was not so simplistic that it laid the blame for all ailments on bad weather. Most illnesses had various degrees of causes and all sorts of variables, including one's lifestyle, could combine to influence what happened in the body.

"MAL ORDEN Y MALA REGLA"—LIFESTYLE

If people felt relatively exposed to one of the main sources of their ailments–the environment—they could at least take solace in the fact that the other major source of sickness—their personal habits—lay somewhat more in their control. It appears, however, that inhabitants of the past were no better than we are today at controlling their unhealthy ways. Agustin Farfán, a sixteenth-century physician who wrote one of the earliest medical guides in New Spain, has trouble containing his annoyance with his contemporaries in his discussion on "weakness of the stomach." "The causes of this illness," he writes, "are many, and the most common is the poor order and regulation [*mal orden y mala regla*] we have in eating and drinking, and if you do not believe me, show me (for the love of God) a man that will desist from eating that which he knows well from experience will do him harm."[44] And, although Cárdenas ascribes much blame to a humid climate, he is equally critical of his fellow creoles for their intemperate ways. The weak stomachs, dropsy, and diarrhea "that afflict everyone and pardon no one" are brought on, in part, by "the little exercise and overindulgence of food and drink that in the Indies people are so accustomed to."[45]

This observation of creole habits was a common one throughout the centuries of Spanish rule, including well into the nineteenth century, when a foreign visitor noted of the upper classes that "the early fading beauty [in the women], the decay of teeth, and the overcorpulency so common amongst them, are no doubt the natural consequences of want of exercise and of injudicious food."[46]

How would *novohispanos* have defined a healthy diet? No easy answer emerges from historical documents; for one thing, unlike the classic ideas on the nature of climate and environment, which were fairly consistent across time and place, ideas on what constituted a proper diet were eclectic. Because diverse foods suited different constitutions and different ages, no standards emerged, except the Hippocratic dictate of moderation in everything. A food such as honey, for example, which was thought to be "choleric" and extremely "hot" in quality, could be harmful to people who were also choleric in temperament and to those who tended to have a lot of natural heat, like the young. In contrast, these same qualities were salubrious to those who were old, phlegmatic in temperament, and to those who were suffering from illnesses caused by an overabundance of phlegm.[47] Additionally, the characteristics of foods were not simply considered in their simple states, they needed to be assessed after they were prepared as well, as different cooking methods—boiling, roasting, or stewing—altered the original qualities of the ingredients. For headaches, one medical guide suggested it was better to eat meats that were roasted, not stewed, whereas lettuce should only be consumed after it was cooked in vinegar and sugar.[48]

Any discussion of diet, too, is complicated by the close connections between medicine and food; in contrast to attitudes today in which a sharp distinction is drawn between prescription drugs and food, early modern societies saw no dividing line between medicines and nourishment. Colonial remedy books are full of food-as-medicine recipes: for bloody diarrhea, Farfán claims that milk "is both medicine and sustenance" (a claim that would cause today's doctors to recoil as dairy products are known to make diarrhea worse!), and that cooked egg yolks "with a bit of mild vinegar" help stop the flow of this "dangerous disease."[49] And, finally, complicating ideas about diet even more is the question of how eating habits were related to social hierarchy—an issue made even murkier in a setting such as New Spain, with its clashing and blending of European and indigenous cultures. Historians have noted that the aristocracy in early modern

Europe—consumers of a meat-rich diet—tended to look down on the culinary practices of the lower orders because they consumed foods, however nourishing, that were generally categorized as animal fodder.[50] Such attitudes took on new meaning in the Americas where Europeans saw much to be desired in the simple diets of the native inhabitants. A recent study noted that the first Spaniards to settle in the Indies "soon bent every effort to bring from Europe the 'civilized' food they longed for." Within a decade or two of the conquests of Mexico and Peru, the essential ingredients for a Mediterranean diet—wheat and barley, wine, eggs, meat, and fowl—were imported abundantly, and, by the end of the sixteenth century, their production, on wheat farms and cattle ranches, was firmly entrenched in the American countryside.[51] Premodern attitudes to diet, therefore, were not as fixed as those people had about the environment; ideas about the consumption of food and drink, and their effect on health were shaped not only by general medical theory, but by cultural factors as well.

Let us begin our inquiry into attitudes about diet with contemporary medical theory. According to the professionals, what happened to food once it entered the body? Their supposition that it provided nourishment for growth and sustenance was not so different from our own, although the mechanics of how this happened do not correspond to modern notions of digestion and metabolism. The Spanish physician Christobal Méndez explained that once food was eaten it went through an elaborate process of digestion:

> [Food] is digested and disposed of four times, and every time it has to be cleaned, modified, and cleared of superfluities. The first time is in the stomach, whence the superfluities go downward to the bowels; the second is in the liver, where the superfluities go to the bile and become what we call spleen; the third is in the veins, whence comes the urine which passes from the kidneys to the bladder; and the fourth is when nutriment is transformed into the substance of our bodies, and from this fourth superfluity are made hair and nails and other superfluities that are disposed of in a sensible way convenient for other things.[52]

Digestion is imagined as an involved and complicated sequence of cleansing and absorption. The "superfluities," however, appear to be a key factor of concern. Méndez explains this further:

> When there are too many superfluities in the body, diseases of repletion appear and kill suddenly. If the superfluities are few and of severe putrefaction, they are followed by fevers, mortal ulcers, rheumatic pains, gout, kidney stones, and mortal indispositions, which although not fatal make life a living death. . . . [Therefore] there must be great regularity in the human body, not only in regard to a proper regime so that

> too many superfluities are not generated, but also in connection with great care and solicitude in expelling them.[53]

Juan de Cárdenas uses the same kind of rationale in pointing out the dangers of overeating, although here "superfluities" become "excrements." The Spanish population of New Spain eats too much, he writes, and this is bad for them because it "generates a large amount of excrements, which suffocate the natural heat [of the body]."[54] Both writers repeatedly identified the excessive eating and drinking habits of their contemporaries as the source of many medical problems.

Agustín Farfán illustrates one way superfluities can harm the body: they do so by thickening the blood so much that it cannot move swiftly though the veins. He singles out creole women who, in his opinion, seem especially prone to this condition because of their laziness and overindulgent habits. Farfán devotes a chapter to the menstruation problems of *criollas*, which according to the doctor was so common that "we see it everyday in maidens, married women, and widows." The main reason for these problems is "the blood, being too thick and too phlegmatic." This affliction was caused by:

> too much eating and too much idleness and too little exercise. These two things the women of New Spain do very well, because at all hours of the day and night one can see them eating delicacies [*golozinas*]. Usually [this is] cacao, eaten and drunk, and this is something they cannot do without. Others overindulge in Chocolate, which is a drink made of many things, among them contrary, thick, and hard to digest. They eat unripe fruit all year long. Others never tire of limes and salt and bitter and sweet oranges. . . . These things thicken the blood and obstruct the veins, as if with stones or mud . . . [55]

Contemporary experts thus believed that gluttony lay at the heart of many illnesses. Too much food and drink produced all sorts of harmful matter that the body simply could not absorb, setting the unsuspecting diner up for trouble later on.

Viewed through the prism of humoral medicine—where bodily fluids, in the right quantity and balance, were of central importance—the human body might be described as a put-through system, absorbing food and expelling wastes. If modern science has persuaded us to see the heart and lungs as crucial organs, the corresponding equivalent for pre-moderns must have been the stomach. Edward Jenner called it the "grand Monarque of the Constitution," and, as a popular English proverb of the time put it: "the belly carries the legs and not the legs the belly."[56] Disorders in other parts of the body were closely connected to what happened in the stomach. Farfán noted that if people would only take care of their stomachs, they would suffer less from other disorders such as gout, *dolor de ijada*, and urinary track problems.[57] In this medical model, in which diseases were not seen as distinct entities but, rather, as temporary concentrations of humors, fluids, or "vapors," pain and malfunction in one area of the body could easily migrate elsewhere. It was essential then that wastes be eliminated efficiently.

Clearing away the superfluities could be done in four ways, wrote Méndez, by "provoking vomiting, bloodletting, purging, and [by giving] something to cause sweating and urination."[58] The idea behind these bedrock therapies of humoralism was that the removal of a bodily fluid—blood, bile, sweat—would release corrupt matter from the body. Among the four humors, the properties of blood were unique; the fluid contained in the veins and arteries was thought to be a mixture of pure blood with small amounts of the other three humors. If nutriment was not digested properly or if excess matter was not excreted in an efficient manner, the vessels of the body would become too full, creating the condition of *plethora*, or an overabundance of blood. The purpose of bloodletting was to diminish a plethora or to remove an excess of one of the other three humors which were present in the blood. Phlebotomy—surely one of the most oft-resorted-to therapies in the history of Western medicine—was employed both therapeutically and prophylactically. Although normally performed by venesection, or the cutting of a vein, in some cases other techniques, such as cupping, applying leeches, cautery, or blistering might be called for.[59]

Vargas Machuca's extensive medical advice for military commanders on the campaign trail surprisingly does not include instructions on how to bleed, even though he recommends this for all fevers. "Where there are no doctors, everyone knows how to bleed," he writes.[60] After reading other manuals describing basic phlebotomy, one wonders how a layman could have managed such a complex, and potentially dangerous, procedure. Alonso López de Hinojosos's book on surgery for the layman includes a whole section on the techniques of bloodletting because it is "of great benefit and great necessity in many towns, mines, and ranches, for the lack of doctors, surgeons, and barbers they have there." His sixteenth-century methods are nearly indistinguishable from those systematized by Galen centuries earlier. His instructions include: how to identify the thirty-three veins—"thirteen in the head, ten in the arms, and eight in the legs"—commonly used for bleeding; how to apply a ligature correctly; and which veins to bleed for specific illnesses.[61] Esteyneffer's *Florilegio medicinal* also contains a detailed tutorial on the art of *sangría*, including how to handle the "timid" patient, or those that tend to faint easily: "if this is from fear (as some are afraid of bleeding) lay them on a bed and wet their face with cold water or delight them by applying things of good odor to their noses . . . and if this is not enough, gently provoke vomiting by placing in the mouth or throat a feather (moistened with oil) . . . after they are feeling comfortable again, give them a bit of soup or a swallow of good wine."[62] Bleeders had to know just how much blood to draw and what side of the body to bleed on. An important strategy in disease treatment was to conduct disturbances in vital parts of the body—the head, the lungs, the liver—to less important areas, a tactic paralleled in the idea of forcing corrupt humors "out" by bringing them to the surface and expelling them through bleeding, purging, or sweating. Similar to bleeding, Esteyneffer often recommended the use of *fuentes*, an opening on the skin made by cautery or incision:

> When the intention is revulsion [*reveler*], or to call the corrupt humor away, then one must open the *fuente* on the opposite part . . . when there is headache caused by a sick liver, then in such a case one must open the fuente in the right leg; and when [the headache] is caused by an indisposition in the spleen, open the fuente in the left leg; and when the pain originates from a sick uterus [*mal de madre*], then it can be opened in any one of the legs.[63]

What emerges from the pages of medical professionals then is that they had fairly elaborate ideas worked out about the processes taking place inside of the body: the constant flow and balance of the four humors, the put-through system needing continual refueling and efficient evacuation of wastes, the various functions of vital organs. But our concern here is with the sufferers themselves. Did lay conceptions about these physiological processes differ so much from medical opinion? Sources from colonial Mexico suggest they did not. This is not to imply that lay people consciously theorized about health and illness; rather that, on some basic level, the assumptions humoralism made about the inner workings of the body were accessible and convincing to people, at least to those whose cultural influences were primarily European. Nor should we suppose that other ideas about disease causation and treatment did not coexist in these same minds. As we have seen elsewhere in this study, empirics of all sorts commonly mixed rational healing strategies with magical and religious methods. But the humoral model was a strong one. Laypeople perfectly understood the need to expel corrupted matter from their bodies when they fell ill, something that is revealed in the countless number of references to the evacuant therapies in contemporary writings. Thus, a sixteenth-century letter writer matter-of-factly relates his experience with an illness that lasted two months in which "they bled me twenty-two times from the arch vein in my right arm, and they purged me four times."[64]

The letters of the Condesa de Miravalle are full of purging and bleeding, her own and of others around her: "I am sorry Maria Antonia still suffers from *reumatismo*," she writes to her son-in-law, "she should be bled"; on another occasion, "the leeches applied to [Maria Antionia's] ankle calmed her down a little"; and when an unnamed friend is ill, she reports: "it seems to be *la gota* [gout], day before yesterday and yesterday he was bleed." The Condesa herself is a firm believer in the power of purges. She uses them both as remedy and prophylaxis—"day after tomorrow I will purge myself"—although she also was frequently bleed: "On Tuesday they applied leeches . . . although I am still ailing"; and, on one occasion, her feet were so swollen from insect bites that "no blood would come out, so they had to bleed me from my arm."[65]

Were people taking great risks when they consented to undergo phlebotomy or drink a strong purge? At least one letter writer saw firsthand the perils of an overly aggressive treatment: "they bleed her six times and because of this she was put in great danger," Juan de Briguega writes about his wife, who, at the time, was seven months pregnant.[66] Although most of the evacuant treatments were probably harmless, the potential hazards of subjecting a patient to excessive bleeding or purging were real because dehydration and serious blood loss could be fatal. General advice cautioned against bleeding pregnant women, small children, the elderly, or the critically ill. It was also thought that venesection should be avoided in hot or cold weather and during a full moon, as the body tended to be at a weaker state during this time.[67] Esteyneffer warned his readers that "violent" purges and vomits, as well as copious bleedings, should always be approached with great prudence. He felt this was especially true in the area of Mexico where he worked in the missions, the far north: "on account of the temperament of these lands, as well as the foods eaten here which do not lend themselves to it, and especially because the Indians [here] are not generally able to stand the bleedings." There were cases, however, when hesitation to bleed should quickly be tossed aside, for example, the onset of a "violent" illness such as "bloody apoplexy, the croup, [the accretion of] phlegm which threatens to suffocate [the patient], and other similarities which clearly need for the blood to be evacuated without any delay whatsoever."[68]

Esteyneffer's intriguing observation that the Indians could not stand the bleedings also was mentioned in a few other sources. The *Relación de Guatulco* states that the Indians had such an aversion to the European practice of bleeding that "they look at it as if it were their death, because they are a weak and gaunt people that do not have the vigor to stand the bleedings." And the Spanish physician Francisco Hernández, in a critique of native doctors, derisively noted that they "never cut anyone's veins," relying instead on diet and simple medicines as their only effective recourse in treating disease.[69] Still, it is not as if Mesoamericans were unfamiliar with drawing blood; the deliberate bleeding of one's self for religious purposes—from the penis, tongue, or ears—was a common prehispanic practice, and Mesoamerican curers frequently relieved swellings by letting off some blood. Headache, for example, was thought to originate from an excess of blood in the head. Sahagún's informants list bleeding as one of the treatments for headache, either by getting the sufferer to sneeze violently enough to cause a nosebleed—through the inhalation of *ecuxo* ("sneeze-plant) or tabacco—or by making a small incision inside the nose with a shape obsidian point. The making of a puncture wound to let blood also was listed as a remedy for swellings in the tongue, nursing women's breasts, and the swellings resulting from broken bones.[70]

But bleeding from the arm, especially for the purposes other than relieving swelling, was undoubtedly a Spanish import. "They did not know what bleeding was, they only used herbs," states the *Relación de Tepuztlan*, while the *Relación de Coatepec* declares that before the conquest the Indians "did not use *sangrías* in their arms; rather, the remedy that they found was to pierce the head, and through the body and chest and belly, with a thin bone, very sharp, or with a snake's fang." Another source says they "punctured themselves with sharp lion and tiger bones, which they believe to be medicinal."[71] Consequently, although bleeding was used in Mesoamerican medicine for some practical purposes, the extensive Galenic practice of phlebotomy, with its rationale so firmly based in the theory of humors, must have been strange (and slightly terrifying!) to Indians in those first contacts with Western medicine, especially because the practice continued to have such strong religious associations for them.

For those colonial Mexicans who monitored their health through a European medical model, then, maintaining a balance of the body's fluids was clearly an important key to wellbeing. Superfluities threatened to upset the balance in numerous ways—by making the blood too thick to flow properly, creating a plethora of blood, or an excess of one of the other humors. As we have seen, overeating was one of the ways that superfluities were generated, and it was for this reason that moderation in diet was prescribed by those who gave medical advice. But what other ideas did people have about the connections between health and the foods they ate? Certainly there were widespread popular beliefs about certain foods and their effects on the body, notions so commonly accepted that they are rarely explained in the historical record. Take fruit, for example, a food that was repeatedly identified as the source of various illnesses and disorders. The *Relaciones Geográficas* mention several times that the cause of disease in Indian towns was the consumption of too much fruit. The *Relación de Cuicatlan*, for example, states that "the diseases they usually have [here] are, for the most part, fevers: because, as this is a hot land, there is much local fruit, and very good, certainly known as the best of New Spain, and because they generally eat these fruits, they tend to get fevers . . ." Another *relación*, says that "this is a town of few sick people and the ones that do fall sick come from eating the local fruit."

We have already seen how the sixteenth-century doctor Farfán rebukes the women of New Spain for eating "green and unripe fruits all year long," including limes and oranges, both bitter and sweet. There also seems to have been similar notions about eating sweets. These same women—again, according to Farfán—"at all hours of the day and many hours of the night" are eating *golozinas*, that is, sweets and delicacies. Nearly two hundred years later, the Condesa de Miravalle is sounding the same kinds of warnings to her daughter's family in Pachuca. During the smallpox epidemic that swept through many parts of New Spain in 1763, she cautions that her grandchildren not be allowed to eat sweets while the threat of smallpox is present; another letter mentions that Maria Antonia's dizzy spells were probably caused by "the sweets she eats."[72] The well-known Doctor Bartolache also cites "the abuse of sweets" as one of the major reasons for the "plague" of *mal histérico*, a condition of the nerves that disproportionately afflicted "people of high or middle category born and educated in a life of leisure [*en el regalo*]."[73]

None of these sources explicitly say why fruit and sweets could be so harmful; apparently, they didn't need to since these beliefs were so commonly accepted. In our own time, similar notions about certain foods and their physiological effects have been, and, in some places still are, accepted as common knowledge: most of us learned at some point in our lives that chocolate causes acne in adolescents and sugar makes small children hyperactive, although double-blinded studies have found no substance to either claim. And yet modern medicine certainly informs our ideas about what constitutes a healthy diet, just as early modern medicine helped shape the concepts people of the past held about their foods. Today's biochemist sees food as a combination of proteins, fats, carbohydrates, vitamins, and other nutrients working in various ways to sustain the body, information that the lay public interprets, in more or less informed ways, as a need to avoid too much fat, eat more fruits and vegetables, and increase their fiber intake. The humoral medical model, which viewed foods in terms of their "qualities," that is, their hot, cold, wet, or dry properties, likewise informed lay ideas about what foods, like fruit and sweets, should be eaten with caution.

Ideas of a proper diet also were closely entangled with the issue of food as an aspect of identity. Class, race, and culture have always influenced notions about eating and drinking, and these are clearly evident in the references both Spaniards and Indians made about each other's culinary practices during the colonial years in Mexico's history. Moreover, European assumptions about foreign lands caused many to question the suitability of New World foods. Because a person's constitution was partly determined by one's native land, a move to a place with different climates, soils, plants and animals could make the foreigner more vulnerable to falling ill. One observer noted that the quality of the food produced in the New World was inferior to that of Europe: "The little virtue and substance of the food in this land shortens one's life . . . a man can eat a variety of these foods, and of these as much as possible and more than normal, and after having eaten he seems to be left with less strength and vigor than before."[74] The Englishman, Thomas Gage, a Dominican friar who traveled through Mexico in the 1620s, makes a similar observation about the food he was served, although he finds it appetizing and delicious.

> . . . in our stomachs we found a great difference between Spain and that country. In Spain and other parts of Europe a man's stomach will hold out from meal to meal, . . . but in Mexico and other parts of America we found that two or three hours after a good meal of three or four several dishes of mutton, veal or beef, kid, turkeys, or other fowls, our stomachs would be ready to faint, and so we were fain to support them with either a cup of chocolate, or a bit of conserve or biscuit, which for that purpose was allowed us in great abundance.

Curious as to why this should be, the inquisitive Gage reports to have found the answer from a "doctor of physic" who told him that the meat lacked nutrition "by reason of the pasture, which is drier and hath not the change of springs" that European pastures have. In addition, the American climate—that ever-powerful force over human bodies—produced things that were "fair outward" but with little substance inside. This reasoning not only applied to meat, fowl, fruits, and vegetables, but to the people there as well.

> Secondly, he told me, the climate of those parts had this effect, to produce a fair shew but little matter or substance. As in the flesh we fed on, so likewise in all the fruits there. These are most fair and beautiful to behold, most sweet and luscious to taste, but have little inward virtue or nourishment at all in them, not half that is in a Spanish *camuesa*, or English Kentish pippin [apple]. And as in meat and fruit there is this inward and hidden deceit, so likewise the same is to be found in the people that are born and bred there, who make fair outward shews, but are inwardly false and hollow-hearted. Which I have heard reported much among the Spaniards to have been the answer of our Queen Elizabeth of England to some that presented unto her of the fruits of America, that surely where those fruits grew, the women were light, and all the people hollow and false-hearted.[75]

Gage's observations about the quality of the foods and peoples of the New World reflect an aspect of the emergent nationalism that was evolving at the time in Europe. Age-old Hippocratic theories about the connections between a peoples' food habits and its geographical location naturally feed into notions of food as a component of group-identity. And because what, and how much, one ate played such a significant role in the delicate balance between sickness and health, the staple diet of Indians—maize and chili, enhanced with a bit of squash, beans, sometimes meat—attracted much comment. The *Relación de Tlaxcala,* for example, states that the illnesses usually acquired by the Indians were caused by an "abundance of choler and phlegm, and other bad humors that they get from their bad diet and lack of proper clothing." A sparse diet was one of the reasons Indians could not tolerate bleedings, another *Relación* observed: the foods and the land did not produce in the local people "a sufficient amount of blood to be drawn."[76] But we should not draw too rigid a picture of European attitudes about the indigenous diet. Juan de Cárdenas praised, at least for health reasons, the way that native Mexicans ate. Because their diet was so healthful—Cárdenas thought chile and maize tortillas helped to cleanse and "dry out" the bad humors from the body—they rarely suffered from such maladies as "rheumatism, *de ijada,* urine or stomach [problems]." Furthermore, the Indian diet contained little meat, at least in comparison with the meat-rich diet of Spaniards, and, most important for Cárdenas, they did not use *manteca,* or lard in their cooking:

> . . . the Spaniards eat all their food or most of it cooked and prepared with *manteca* instead of oil, and since the *manteca* of pork is extremely phlegmatic, from there follows many rheumatisms, which the Indians will never suffer from because they will never allow food to be cooked with *manteca* in their house, nor with any other thing except chili or salt.[77]

Although wheat was grown in New Spain, wine and olive oil—the other two essentials in the holy trinity of the Mediterranean diet—were never successfully produced in the colony. Although no universally accepted substitute for wine ever emerged, creoles readily adapted to the use of lard in their cuisine, a practice initially condemned by the Indians. In her book on the prehispanic culinary practices of the Aztec, Maya, and Inca cultures, Sophie Coe notes that native Americans found the idea of eating animal fat repulsive, so much so, in fact, that cooking with lard was noted by the Indians as one of the main horrors brought by the Spanish, ranking alongside beatings and prisons. (In time, however, they discovered that the addition of a bit of manteca to tamales made them fluffier and more delicate.)[78]

Spaniards enthusiastically embraced one native Mexican food, however, and in doing so were key players in introducing the rest of the world to a culinary pleasure we all take for granted today. That food was chocolate, made from the seeds of the *cacao* tree, or *Theobroma cacao,* as it came to be called by the Swedish naturalist Linnaeus in the eighteenth century. Cacao was first domesticated by the Olmec and Maya peoples in that area of Mesoamerica that contains the natural habitat of cacao trees, the tropical rain forests. By the time that the Spanish conquered Mexico, cacao had become an esteemed product among the Nahua-speaking peoples of central Mexico, serving both as currency and beverage, although its consumption appears to have been confined to the Aztec elite.[79] Both Native Americans and early modern Europeans believed that cacao had medicinal benefits. The *Florentine Codex* lists chocolate as an ingredient in cures for stomach pain, diarrhea, and "the spitting of blood." Among the treatments described in the *Badianus Manuscript* is the use of cacao flowers to perfume a bath recommended for curing fatigue. And Francisco Hernández, who, in consultation with native doctors, carried out the first thorough study of Mexican medicinal plants, noted that cacao was prescribed to patients suffering from fever and liver problems. The Nahuas also apparently believed that chocolate, especially in its green or unroasted form, could intoxicate its drinker: "when much drunk . . . [it] makes one drunk, takes effect on one, makes one dizzy, confuses one, makes one sick, deranges one." But when used with proper moderation, it "gladdens one, refreshes one, consoles one, invigorates one."[80]

That Europeans were crazy for this drink is clearly evident from the abundance of contemporary writing devoted to it. Undoubtedly this popularity stemmed from the perception that it provided nutrition, had great medicinal properties, and, at the same time, was extremely pleasurable to drink. In contrast to the social prohibitions that limited its availability in precontact times, colonial authorities did not affix any particular social meanings to its use, thus chocolate consumption in New Spain was a daily practice for most social groups. On his visit from Spain in the second half of the eighteenth century, the friar Francisco Ajofrín was amazed at the ubiquity and frequency of this Mexican ritual:

> The use of chocolate in all of America is very frequent; the most moderate person has it twice a day, in the morning and at three o'clock in the afternoon; many have it three times; not a few, four times, and some even more. In the morning and even in the afternoon the maids and servants, the coachmen, the attendants, blacks, and mulattos all drink it; it is so common that even the muleteers, shoemakers, officials and all classes of people use it in the afternoon and in the morning.[81]

The frequent use of chocolate had spread to native communities by the end of the sixteenth century, a fact verified by the native informants in the *Relación de Guatulco*, who lamented the ubiquity of this practice by linking it to contemporary afflictions. In their minds, the consumption of cacao and "other mixed brews" went hand-in-hand with eating the "heavy foods" of the Spaniards, a practice that "made their bodies heavy" and led to sickness and shortened lives.[82]

The supposed medicinal qualities of cacao certainly excited the European imagination. Chocolate was not the only American product to do so—tobacco, sarsaparilla, and guaiacum were just a few of the other new plants to accumulate fantastic claims of curing power to their names. But because cacao, with its swelling popularity as a food and drink, was undoubtedly consumed by many more people than any other American elixir, it quickly sparked a vigorous debate about its effects on the human body. Of course, it was viewed from the start in the context of humoral pathology and therapeutics. Hernández wrote that the cacao seed had a "cool" nature; thus, drinks made from it were good in hot weather and helpful to patients suffering from fever and ailments of the liver. He also noted, as did other commentators later on, that chocolate had properties that made its drinker "extraordinarily fat" if drunk frequently; this made it useful in treating the "thin and weak" patient. Juan de Cárdenas, too, wrote extensively about chocolate in his treatise on New Spain. He argued that untoasted cacao was harmful when taken in its simple, raw form: among other things, it could constrict the belly, obstruct menstruation and urination, make one short of breath, and "cause and generate perpetual anxiety and melancoly." If toasted, ground, and mixed with *atole* (ground maize and water), however, it was extremely nourishing, and a potent remedy for all sorts of "obstructions," female problems (*mal de madre*), in addition to brightening one's mood.[83]

The Dominican friar Thomas Gage relished his chocolate, which he drank several times a day because, as we have already seen, his stomach often was "faint" from hunger. He attributed his good health during his stay in the Indies to this habit: "and with this custom I lived twelve years in those parts healthy, without any obstructions or oppilations, not knowing what either ague or fever was." During the seventeenth century, after its use had widely radiated throughout Spain, even more fantastical claims were made about chocolate's panacean qualities. Perhaps Antonio Colmenero de Ledesma's *Curioso tratado de la naturaleza y calidad del chocolate* best typifies the excessive optimism some Europeans had for cacao:

> . . . [chocolate] vehemently incites to Venus, and causeth conception in women, hastens and facilitates their delivery; it is an excellent help to digestion, it cures consumptions, and the cough of the lungs, the New Disease, or plague of the guts, and other fluxes, the green sickness, jaundice, and all manner of inflammations and obstructions. It quite takes away the morpheus, cleaneth the teeth and sweetneth the breath, provokes urine, cures the stone, and expels poison, and preserves from all infectious diseases.[84]

Colmenero de Ledesma's claims that chocolate was some sort of miracle nostrum, curing everything from infertility to kidney stones and bad breath, may seem like nothing more than sensationalist hype. But when viewed in the context of the seventeenth century, an age when contemporary therapies had little efficacy, this almost naive optimism about a new medicine reminds us once again that the threat of disease and disability intruded into daily life in a way that would be hard to imagine in the age of modern medicine. Not everyone agreed that chocolate was a new panacea, however. Farfán, as already noted, found its frequent use deleterious and blamed all sorts of ills on its "abuse." Grounding his objections in classical medicine, he noted that it was made of many "contrary" things and was "thick and difficult to digest." In the eighteenth century, Bartolache made similar claims about the harmful consequences of chocolate drinking; "people of moderate circles and the poor" were especially prone to these ill effects, as they were forced to buy chocolate of questionable quality that contained "certain drugs and ingredients that are extremely damaging to their health." Gage also reports that he has "known some that have been the worse for it, either for drinking it with too much sugar, which hath relaxed their stomachs, or for drinking it too often."[85]

European women quickly noticed the cosmetic properties of cacao. Over half the weight of the shelled and degermed cacao bean is made up of fat, or "cacao butter," a product, Gage noted, "I have seen drawn out . . . by the Creole women for to oint their faces."[86] But face cream was not the only cosmetic use women made of cacao. Several sources mention that women in New Spain ate cacao in its solid form because they believed that it altered the coloring of their faces. This strange practice was not limited to eating cacao, but also included eating "*barro*" or "*tierra*," that is, clay or earth, usually in the form of "earthenware, as pots or pieces of lime walls." Gage wrote that eating cacao in this manner, "as many Creole and Indian women eat it," made them "look of a broken, pale, and earthly color," a fashion that was much "used among the Spanish women" who believed that this facial coloring "well becomes them." This quest for "*color de damas*," or paleness in the face was vigorously condemned by Cárdenas, who claimed this caused menstrual problems in the women who practiced this "vice" by thickening the blood and causing obstructions.

> . . . this vice of eating *tierra*, *barro*, *cacao*, and other similar filth . . . which are made up of thick, terrestrial, and feculent things, causes terrible closures and blockages in the veins. But if asked why are the women of this land [New Spain] more given to eating earth and cacao than women in different provinces, I would respond that some do it for pure vice, pretending only to bring about a broken color [*traer quebrado el color*], (which they call ladies' color).[87]

Along with the overindulgence of sweets, chocolate, and fruit, Farfán adds eating "*tierra de adobes*" to his list of vices committed by the Spanish women of

New Spain. These women "do not leave a colored jar's lid, nor the jar itself, uneaten. And if this were only the young girls, I would not be so disturbed, but it's the ones with a head full of gray hair that are the most licentious and disorderly [*viciosas y desregladas*].[88]

Today, this odd habit of clay-eating would certainly be diagnosed by the modern practitioner as pica, the term given to "the compulsive consumption of substances not generally considered food." Modern research has shown, both historically and cross-culturally, that those most prone to pica are young children, pregnant women, the mentally retarded, and people with mental disorders. The kinds of items usually consumed also seem to be consistent across time and cultures; these include, coal, ice, chalk, plaster, and various types of earth, especially clay. The consumption of the latter, sometimes called geophagy or geophagia, a Greek term meaning "earth-eating," is the most commonly noted type of pica, and some researchers today believe that it may be a response to fill a nutritional deficiency, such as low iron or calcium.[89] Clay consumption can lead to several health problems, however, such as liver and kidney damage, constipation, abdominal problems, mercury poisoning, and anemia.

This last complication may help explain the cosmetic reason women in New Spain took to eating their clay pots: people with anemia become quite pale. The ideal standards of feminine beauty at this time were fairly uniform across national borders in Europe and remained virtually unchanged throughout the sixteenth, seventeenth, and eighteenth centuries. For the face, the aesthetic canon dictated that the skin be creamy white, lips and cheeks painted red, black eyebrows, and blond hair. Just a causal glance at some of the portraits painted of elite families in eighteenth-century Mexico confirms that European standards of feminine beauty were vigorously adhered to on this side of the Atlantic. Topped with fair-haired wigs, these creole and Spanish women are heavily powdered and rouged, presenting faces of porcelain perfection to their observers. What a contrast to the images of women depicted in the *pinturas de castas*, where racial mixing has progressively darkened skin and hair as one moves further away from European blood "purity."[90] The colonial practice of eating *barro y tierra*, then, clearly reminds us that the culturally-bound connections between diet, fashion, and health are not only features of the modern era, but have been shaping human lives for a long time.

Although it did not create as much commentary as chocolate consumption, indigenous lifestyle was also a topic that generated questions about human health. Because the native population of Mexico suffered disproportionately from epidemics and general hardship during Spanish rule, anyone today delving into colonial Mexican sources comes across a range of contemporary opinion on Indians' daily-life habits. These opinions have been scrutinized by modern scholars to show how the Spanish attempted to make sense of the

Mesoamerican world by using, not surprisingly, their own "European grids and vocabularies."[91] For our purposes here these opinions likewise help to illuminate general conceptions the European (and the ever-expanding Europeanized) population had about health and lifestyle. This comes through especially on comments, not only about indigenous diet but also on the manner of dress, patterns of work, and other practices such as bathing. In many of the *Relaciones Geográficas,* which offer a mixture of indigenous statements and Spanish transcription (and interpretation), we hear a variety of explanations as to why inhabitants of Indian towns became ill. Geography and climate, as we have already seen, were critical factors in a locale's salubrity, but lifestyle—and especially the change from a precontact lifestyle to one modified by Spanish customs—is mentioned frequently as well. In this diversity of explanations, perhaps it is worthwhile to try to distinguish Spanish voices from those of the Indians.

One detects immediately a European view in the strong aversion to the idleness, laziness, and drunkenness that many observers saw in native towns. "The Indians here are extremely fond of the wine of Castile, which they buy for a high price . . . And because they spend so much on drink, they have very little money," states the *Relación de Cuahuitlan.* Another blames the "many pestilences" for the horrible decline in native population, but also "the idleness and laziness of the Indians, because they do not work as much as they used to."[92] The priest Cayetano de Cabrera y Quintero, whose book, *Escudo de armas,* commemorated the end of the horrible epidemic of *matlazáhuatl* that ravaged New Spain between 1736 and 1738, cited four major reasons why so many Indians died of pestilence. In addition to the extreme temperature changes in Mexico City—"hot during the day, cold at night (and much more for those with insufficient clothing, and no other habits but drinking)"—was the abuse of alcohol, the poor diet (both quality and quantity of food) and "drinking cold water while sweating." For Cabrera y Quintero, however, drinking was the biggest culprit. The Indians were especially vulnerable to epidemic diseases because of their "abuse and excess of counterfeit *aguardientes, tepaches* [pulque mixed with sugar and other substances], and other fermented drinks. The same is true of *aguardiente de Castilla* [Spanish brandy], no matter how good it is . . . it should also be noted that [they often] get drunk on pulque contaminated with harmful twigs and herbs, which they use to fortify it."[93]

This Spanish preoccupation with native drinking, which has been skillfully explored by William Taylor, points to basic cultural differences in the way Indians and Spaniards viewed the consumption of alcoholic beverages. Inheritors of a Mediterranean culture that recognized wine as one of its most valued symbols of civilization and Catholic heritage, Spaniards considered wine an essential ingredient to a proper meal but outward signs of drunkenness as barbaric. With wine occupying such a central position in Spanish culture, not to mention the importance humoralism gave to moderation in general, it is not hard to see why Spaniards, desperate to explain the decline of the indigenous population, would attribute the (in their view) misuse of alcohol as a major cause of disease. The Indians, however, did not hold the same ideals of drinking; their colonial practices, as Taylor shows, were derived from centuries-long traditions of ritual drinking. Moderation—undoubtedly the most important ideal guiding personal behavior in precontact society—was defined in terms of how often, not how much. Periodic heavy drinking, according to occasion, was the norm, with no shame attached to showing intoxication; daily, solitary drinking, as that practiced by the Spaniards, was considered an inappropriate use of alcohol.[94] But there is little doubt that the breakdown of prehispanic social structure, which had limited access to alcohol with rigid social norms, and the opportunity to make money in the colonial economy, led to more drinking in Indian towns. While traveling in Guatemala, Thomas Gage noted that many of "the baser and poorer sort" of Spaniards there unduly exploited the Indians' love of drink by selling them watered-down wine for high prices and then robbing them once they were drunk.[95]

The native Mexicans who served as informants to the *Relaciones Geográficas* saw the causes of mortality in the same kinds of things as their Spanish transcribers, albeit with less inclination to moralize in European terms. But they were also more prone to see the state of native decline in terms of acculturation as a whole, a loss of a way of life, and the collapse of standards that had previously given structure and meaning to the community. What emerges as a theme in many of the *relaciones* is that austerity, frugality and demanding work are linked to a longer and healthier life. Precontact life was healthier, many reasoned, because then the Indians were "more accustomed to work than now . . . the greater convenience [*el regalo*] they have now is the cause of their illnesses."[96] The principle reason for so much illness today, states another *relación*:

> is that before they made them work very hard, they never let them be idle for one moment, and they slept on a plank, and now they are often idle and they work little, and when they do work, it is by force and they are berated and threatened, and it is already mid-day when they go out to work.[97]

One historian has noted the paradoxical element in this analysis: the hardships of a former existence seem to be associated with a better quality of life, whereas the supposed "benefits" of material acculturation under Spanish rule—the introduction of European clothing, more meat in the diet, raised beds, tables and chairs, and a lasting peace to Central Mexico, which ended the continual need for military recruits—are linked to the incomprehensible decline in native population. In these native sketches of precontact existence—the old way of life that by this time, the 1580s, was probably more stereotyped, even idealized, than real—and colonial life, one senses the word *trabajo*, much used in these accounts, has two different meanings for the native informants: a prehispanic notion of "work" as "a cluster of activities, regulated, organized by the traditional authority and even including war" compared to its colonial meaning as an oppressive task.[98] The informants in the *Relación de Epazoyuca* bring these distinct notions of work to life by juxtaposing activity in prehispanic times—the "running and jumping," clearly a reference to training for warfare—and the forced work in the mines under Spanish taskmasters. Epazoyuca is located in the present-day state of Hidalgo, a site of lucrative silver mines in colonial times:

> Now they are becoming delicate, because, in former times they exercised in many tasks, slept in the streets, and went around nude to the cold and sun. They exercised in running and jumping, and they did not all leave the pueblo, only the great ones who went to war where the authorities sent them, even if it was to remote places. And now they do not live as long, because they are overworked as porters [*tamemes*] and occupied in many things, and in service to the mines; because they [are forced to leave] their natural place, to eat wet tortillas and to sleep on humid ground . . . For these reasons they are greatly suffering, and they are sick and they live a short time.[99]

Many of the Indians that served as informants to the *Relaciones Geográficas*, then, sought explanations for the demographic loss by comparing life before and after the coming of the Spaniards. What was lost, in their view, was a way of life, a totality of customs and practices that kept them alert, agile, and healthy.

Another indigenous practice that generated a fair amount of Spanish commentary was bathing. To the sixteenth-century Iberian, frequent bathing, or the deliberate immersion of one's body in water, was to needlessly place one's health in peril. Native Mexicans, in contrast, had inherited very different notions about water's affect on the body and high standards of personal cleanliness were common in Mesoamerican society. With the exception of some individuals—certain priests, for instance, who for ritualistic reasons could not wash—most Nahuas bathed daily, and even used soap made from the fruit of the *copalxóctl* plant. In addition, bathing, as has already been noted, was an important therapeutic practice, especially the use of the *temazcal*, or steam bath. Bathing rituals also clearly held religious meanings for the Indians since divine intervention was such an inseparable part of native curing methods. Undoubtedly, Spaniards were troubled by this native practice, not only because they suspected it kept alive a significant part of native religious devotion but also because it fell outside their norms of civilized medicine. Several of the *Relaciones* mention it as a source of Indian illness. The *Relacion de Uexutla* states that "the natives bathe a lot, and because of this, many die." Likewise the Indians of *Citlaltomagua*, an *estancia* in the colonial jurisdiction of Acapulco, suffer from "many diseases," because they are "very disorderly, without any order in their illnesses, which causes many of them to die." This informant's critique of native medical practices centered on their therapeutic use of the bath:

> [When] they have fever, which is the most common illness they have, they go to the river and bathe, which, having fever, they become sick from the chill [*pasmo*] or they suddenly get *dolor de costado*, from which they die without even knowing which disease they had; or if they have a contagious disease, like *bubas*, or smallpox or measles, right away they are headed for the river to bathe, because their cure is bathing . . . and after giving birth, the Indian women go to the river and bathe, even when they are menstruating, and for this reason they do not live as long as people in other *provincias*.

The author of this passage unequivocally links the "chilling" of the wet body to sickness, a linkage that the natives do not seem to share. The climate in *Citlaltomagua* is hot which intensifies the chill; the Indians do not understand this danger so that when "they bathe, they are chilled and many die of *pasmo* without understanding the *pasmo*."[100]

Why did Spaniards see such a health risk in bathing? Our earlier examination of climate and health revealed an early modern Europe anxious about the frailty of the bodily shell. Porous and permeable, the skin was easily breached by heat and water, allowing a myriad of harmful substances to slip into the body. The author of one sixteenth-century health manual listed some of the hazards of bathing: it depletes one's energy and overheats the body; it sometimes causes fainting and provokes vomiting; and it forces the bad humors to descend, disturbing and moving them about. If one must bathe, certain rules had to be observed. No baths for at least three hours after eating, unless one wants to become fat, as some very "thin and dry" men do. Because excessive sweating during bathing could be harmful, adding small quantities of cold water and moistening the skin with oil is recommended. Above all, one should not remain in the water too long. The author of this book, who was writing specifically for the courtier class that attended the royal court of Charles V in the 1520s, believed that Spaniards were not well suited for frequent bathing. They were not used to it, he writes, therefore it would not be beneficial to them, except in times of illness. Consequently, the only appropriate way for Spaniards to bathe is "from the knees down."[101]

Immersion in water, therefore, involved a calculated risk; the bath had to be tailored to the season, time of day, the individual's temperament, sex, and state of health. These beliefs had implications for contemporary concepts of cleanliness. Our own insistence on bodily cleanliness—that is, a body without bodily smells—might lead us to believe that people of the early modern era did not have similar values. The French historian, Georges Vigarello, has shown this was not the case, at least not for court society in sixteenth- and seventeenth-century Europe. Cleanliness mattered, but it was attached almost exclusively to one's linen and outward appearance; the body, deeply hidden beneath layers of clothing, mattered less. Nor does it appear that early moderns were any less aware of the need to remove certain odors from their bodies then we are, but they assumed friction and perfume, not washing, was the way to do this. Personal daily grooming, at least for the elite classes, consisted of carefully cleansing the visible areas of the body, the hands and face, and the "dry wash" of those hidden regions of the body which generated offensive odors. Here is Christobal Mendez's version of a proper daily toilette:

> . . . the face should be washed with cold water, the eyes cleaned of the slimy humor which runs from the eyes, and with the little finger clean the nostrils and ears very clear, and move them very much inside, wash teeth and mouth very well with water, and if it is possible wash the eyes, if a youth with rosewater, and if an old man with wine. Both of them should take two swallows of water and gargle very gently. If there is sunshine look toward it and sneeze. Afterwards take a root of the walnut tree and clean the teeth with it and also with a little bit of myrrh, which brings great benefit to them. And before all this while still in bed ask for a little aromatic wine, wet a piece of wool in it, and rub under the arms with it, in the lower parts and between the toes which moreover is great cleanliness and a very beneficial medicine.

But what is a person to do after physical activity has left the body sweaty and sticky? For this Mendez recommends, "if it is not too cold," that the individual take off his shirt and "rub the body in every way possible with some rough cloth, rubbing the arms downward and the legs and all the rest." Afterward, he should anoint his face and wrists with aromatic water and then put on a clean shirt that has been "smoked with some good fragrance—the best and healthiest is rosemary."[102] These older notions of cleanliness, which applied solely to the visible parts of the body, the hands and face, and to the linen peeping out from men's doublets and women's dresses, began changing at the very end of the eighteenth century, first in the upper classes and later in their imitators, the emerging middle classes. By the nineteenth century, a new understanding emerged about the body and the effects of water, and new texts on hygiene—now focused on the hazards of dirt—began to describe the benefits of cleaning with water and the use of soap.[103]

What we learn from this brief examination of the ideas people had about the connections between the environment, daily lifestyle, and their health is that the body's internal workings were most easily affected by what one ate or drank, the quality of the air, and the temperatures one was exposed to. In the commentary of ordinary people and the advice of professionals, these were the issues which seemed to generate the most concern. But other aspects of the nonnaturals occasionally are mentioned as well. Common sense notions about sleeping patterns were explained within the humoral framework: too much sleep was unhealthy because "it increased the harmful humors, especially those in the head," but lack of sleep also had repercussions for health as it tended to deplete the good humors in the body. The most common fear about sleeping seemed to be its coming too soon after a meal. One should never sleep directly after eating, says one advice manual, "because from this comes much harm, such as gout, cough, headache, and many other diseases." Christobal Mendez thought that one should resist sleeping after the midday meal, as "many rheumatisms and even very persistent colds" come from this practice: "it occurs that as soon as one has eaten there comes a great tendency to sleep, but if you stand up, it is soon forgotten and that is beneficial."[104]

The importance of adequate exercise also was mentioned at times by early modern authors of health manuals. This is somewhat surprising, as the idea that exercise plays a key part in preventive medicine strikes most of us as an exclusively modern phenomenon, especially now that health clubs, exercise machines, and personal trainers have become such a routine part of everyday life. But a concern with the body's "movement and rest" was an important component of classical hygiene, one of the six non-naturals elaborated by the founders of Western medicine. As we have already noted many times in this chapter, idleness, that bane of the leisure classes, was cited as one of the reasons for ill health among the European population of New Spain. Both Farfán and Cárdenas, our sixteenth-century commentators on creole lifestyles, decried the *mucho ocio y poco ejercicio* they saw in their contemporaries.[105]

Today, we know that physical activity is beneficial because it burns excess calories, improves the cardiovascular system, and increases bone density. Given the prominent role that food and the stomach played in the humoral conception of the body, it is not surprising to find that the most common rationale early moderns had for exercising was as an aid to digestion. Christobal Mendez, the author of one of the first books written on exercise in early modern Europe, advocated exercising because it increased the "natural heat" of the body which made "digestion greater and more perfect and pour[ed] throughout the body that which is necessary to preserve health." It also helped rid the body of "superfluities," that dangerous build-up of bad humors that threatened to tip the balance toward sickness. Assuming that these authors did not envision exercise to include such things as swimming laps or aerobic classes, what exactly did they mean by the word *ejercicio?* Of all the medical advice perused here, only Mendez elaborates; for him, exercise includes walking, hunting, horseback riding, bowling, dancing, playing games such as horseshoes, quoits, throwing *barras* or spears, shooting arrows, fencing, or playing swords with both hands. Of course, some of these—the "games with arms, hunting, and breaking horses"—are only advisable "for strong men." More suitable for "delicate men" or "men of letters, religion, and other similar professions," was the moderate exercise of walking. For women, Mendez also recommends regular physical activity: "Since many ladies go hunting, why cannot a lady bowl with enjoyment in her hall, and with other ladies, or secluded (where no one sees them) or dance whenever the opportunity?"[106] Obviously, Mendez's advice was intended for the small elite classes of sixteenth-century Spain who enjoyed the leisure of being able to pursue these kinds of activities. We also must keep in mind that then, as today, advice books were prescriptive texts rather than accurate reflections of how people actually lived or thought. Nevertheless, this early treatise on the benefits of exercise, which links lifestyle and physical well-being in a way that, apart from its humoral interpretation, would make sense to today's reader, illustrates the importance a preventative health regime played in early modern medical theory, which, in turn, informed the commonsense notions of a lay public.

Another one of the six nonnaturals, the body's evacuations and retentions, was concerned not only with the quantity, quality, and regularity of the removal of bodily wastes but also with sexual intercourse because this involved (especially for men) the loss of a bodily fluid. Mendez likens both sex and defecating to an act of nature that "expels something superfluous" from the body. Just as the "sort of comfort" one has "when something is expelled in the lower pathways," so, too, "the pleasure found during the joining of male and female is in great part due to what is expelled which is superfluity not needed in the body." We have seen repeatedly throughout this chapter just how significant bodily evacuations were in early modern medicine, not only in terms of reading the body for signs of illness, but as mainstay therapies as well. It is not surprising, therefore, that the sexual act would generate a variety of medical opinion.

Take, for example, Luis Lobera de Avila's advice to the gentlemen of the Spanish court in the sixteenth century, whose compendium of health advice includes a chapter on the potential "harms and benefits of coitus." One should never engage in coitus, he writes, if they are "phlegmatic, nor if they are replete with wine or drunk; nor when they emerge from the bath, nor if they have diarrhea, nor after a bleeding, nor after hard work." He recommends the use of certain foods to increase one's "vigor and semen," such as eggs, chicken livers, partridges, and a good, heavy red wine," and, as a further precaution, he urges men to always carry with them "things that smell good and are aromatic." As in all other aspects of the humoral framework, moderation here, too, was the key: too much sex could damage the nerves and the eyes, deplete one's strength, and "in a short time make men old," whereas a more moderate sex life "relieves the body, alleviates the head and understanding and cures some diseases." This humoral emphasis on sexual moderation is very reminiscent of the Nahua elders' exhortations that a too-vigorous carnal life will drain a man of his strength, causing him to become dry and shriveled before his time. Sex, of course, had to bear much more moral weight than other bodily practices and that comes through in some of the medical advice. Agustín Farfán, a doctor who later entered the Augustinian order, has strong words for those men who are so "unrestrained" in their sexual appetites that they must engage in sex right after a meal, since there "is nothing that damages and destroys the stomach and body more than these acts committed on a full stomach." He likens such men to "course brutes in the countryside" and warns that children produced in these matings are likely to be weak and sickly.[107]

One of the central arguments to emerge from this study is that unless they lived in isolated indigenous villages—a condition that declined in the eighteenth century significantly—most laypeople in colonial Mexico held ideas about medicine that were not so different from those of the professionals. This is because the separation between learned and domestic medicine had not yet solidified into the two distinct spheres that were later to emerge in the nineteenth and twentieth centuries. The tenets of good hygiene, or as the medical books called them, the nonnaturals, formed the bedrock of humoraliam, the medical framework introduced to Mexico by the Spanish Conquest, providing a means by which laypeople could conceptually gain access to medical ideas, especially because hygiene's concern was with everyday lifestyle and one's relationship to the environment. The argument here is not that the rules of hygiene were followed by everyone; on the contrary, we have seen from the colonial sources that have formed the basis of this chapter that they were not. But an examination of the commentary on preventive medicine offers us a glimpse of how people explained why they became ill or how they thought they might avoid disease. Furthermore, a look at this prosaic yet essential aspect of daily life through the particular historical lens of colonial Mexico, enhances our understanding of how Europeans made sense of the foreignness of America. For Spaniards and their cultural contemporaries, the creoles, the medical framework of humoralism—in its essence, a rational explanation of the relationship between the physicality of human beings and the material conditions in which they lived—provided them with a way to judge the new foods, climates, and peoples of their dominions across the Atlantic.

NOTES

1. AMRT *Miravalles*, 21 de julio, 1757; RG, Vol. II, p.168; Antonio de Ciudad Real, *Tratado curioso y docto de las grandezas de la Nueva España*, ed. Josefina García Quintana and Victor M. Castillo Farreras (México: UNAM, 1993), Vol. II, pp. 389–90.

2. Vivian Nutton, "Humoralism," in CEHM, Vol. I, p. 281; Roy Porter, *The Greatest Benefit to Mankind: A Medical History of Humanity* (New York: W.W. Norton & Company, 1997), pp. 56–7.

3. Nancy G. Siraisi, *Medieval & Early Renaissance Medicine: An Introduction to Knowledge and Practice* (Chicago: University of Chicago Press, 1990), p. 106.

4. Nutton, p. 283.

5. Quoted in Andrew Wear, "The History of Personal Hygiene," in CEHM, Vol. I, p. 1288.

6. Nutton, p. 289.

7. Ibid., p. 286; Porter, *The Greatest Benefit to Mankind*, p. 60.

8. Nutton, pp. 288–90.

9. Ibid., p. 290.

10. Juan de Esteyneffer, *Florilegio medicinal de todas las enfermedades*, 2 vols., ed. Ma. Del Carmen Anzures y Bolaños (México: Academia Nacional de Medicina, 1978), Vol. I, pp. 146–7.

11. Wear, pp. 1283–4.

12. Ibid., p. 1290.

13. Christobal Mendez, *Book of Bodily Exercise* (New Haven, CT: Elizabeth Licht, 1960), pp. 64–7.

14. Juan de Cárdenas, *Problemas y secretos maravillosos de las Indias* (Madrid: Alianza Editorial, 1988), p. 204.

15. Ibid., pp. 205, 214–15.

16. Caroline Hannaway, "Environment and Miasmata," in CEHM, Vol. I pp. 292–3.

17. RG, Vol. II., p. 104.

18. RG, Vol. VI, p. 240.

19. PNE, pp. 245–6.

20. Ibid., p. 76.

21. "Antonio Mateos a su hijo Antonio Mateos, en Alcuéscar," Valle de Tlaxcala, miércoles de ceniza, 1561(?), in Enrique Otte, *Cartas privadas de emigrantes a Indias* (México: Fondo de Cultura Económica, 1996), pp. 144–5.

22. "Bartolomé de Morales a su padre Antón Pérez, en Sevilla," México, 30.X.1573, in Otte, pp. 72–3.

23. RG, Vol. I, p. 42.

24. D. Bernardo de Vargas Machuca, *Milicia y descripción de Las Indias* (Madrid. Librería de Victoriano Suarez, 1892), Vol. I, p. 130.

25. Juan de Cárdenas, p. 87.

26. Ibid., p. 88.

27. Ibid., pp. 37–42.

28. Ibid., pp. 216 and 206.

29. Ibid., p. 91.

30. Ciudad Real, Vol. II, p. 314.

31. Pedro Arias de Benavides, *Secretos de cirugía* (México: Academia Nacional de Medicina, 1992), p. 45.

32. RG, Vol. V, p. 317.

33. P. Fray Francisco de Ajofrín, *Diario del viaje . . .* , 2 vols. (Madrid: Archivo Documental Español, 1958), Vol. I, p. 36.

34. Andrew Wear, p. 1291; see also Michael Worboys, "Tropical Diseases," in CEHM, Vol. I, pp. 512–36.

35. *Las Gaceta de México*, miércoles 24 de marzo, Vol. I, no. 5, pp. 46, 55–6.

36. Hannaway, pp. 296–300.

37. Roy Porter and Dorothy Porter, *In Sickness and in Health: The British Experience* (London: Croom Helm, 1987), pp. 158–9.

38. Martha Eugenia Rodríguez, *Contaminación e insalubridad en la ciudad de México en el siglo XVIII* (México: Departamento de Historia y Filosofía de la Medicina, Facultad de Medicina/ UNAM, 2000), p. 26.

39. Hannaway, p. 295.

40. Rodríguez, p. 23.

41. Cited in Rodríguez, pp. 27 and 34.

42. Alain Corbin, *The Foul and the Fragrant: Odor and the French Social Imagination* (Leamington Spa, UK: Berg Publishers, 1986), pp. 22–3.

43. José Ignacio Bartolache, *Mercurio Volante* (México: UNAM, 1983), p. 199; Esteyfenner, Vol. I, pp. 502–03; Rodríguez, pp. 28–9; Mendez, p. 8; Luis Lobera de Avila, *Banquete de nobles caballeros* (Madrid: Reimpresiones Bibliograficas, 1952), p. 153, 149; Porter and Porter, p. 159.

44. Fray Agustín Farfán, *Tractado breve de medicina* (Madrid: Ediciones Cultura Hispanica, 1944), p. 2.

45. Cárdenas, p. 240–3.

46. MME. Calderon de la Barca, *Life in Mexico, During a Residence of Two Years in that Country* (New York: E.P. Dutton and Co., 1946), p. 99.

47. Cárdenas, p. 89.

48. Esteyneffer, Vol. I, pp. 160–1.

49. Farfán, pp. 16–17.

50. Pelling, *The Common Lot*, p. 46.

51. Arnold J. Bauer, *Goods, Power, History. Latin America's Material Culture*, (Cambridge: Cambridge University Press, 2001), pp. 63–9.

52. Mendez, p. 21.

53. Ibid.

54. Cárdenas, p. 249.

55. Farfán, p. 34.

56. Both cited in Porter and Porter, p. 47.

57. Farfán, p. 3.

58. Mendez, p. 22.

59. Harold J. Cook, "Physical Methods," in CEHM, Vol. II, pp. 941–3.

60. Vargas Machuca, Vol. I, p. 130.

61. Alonso López de Hinojosos, *Suma y recopilación de cirugía con un arte para sangrar muy útil y provechosa* (México: Academia Nacional de Medicina, 1977), pp. 95–107.

62. Esteyneffer, Vol. II, p. 729.

63. Esteyneffer, Vol. II, p. 716.

64. "Hernán Ruiz a su mujer Mariana de Montedoca en Sevilla" México, 21.X. 1584, in Otte, pp. 108–9.

65. AMRT Miravalles, 2 de junio, 1760; 19 de febrero, 1759; 9 de mayo, 1757; 4 de abril, 1757; 9 de agosto,1762; 28 de agosto, 1759; 10 de julio, 1760.

66. "Juan de Briguega a su hermano Pedro Garcia, en Brihuega," 16.1.1572, in Otte, p. 154.

67. Linda E. Voigts and Michael R. McVaugh, eds., *A Latin Technical Phlebotomy and its Middle English Translation: Transactions of the American Philosophical Society*, 1984, Vol. 74, pt. 2, pp. 5 and 56.

68. Esteyneffer, pp. 150 and 148.

69. RG, Vol. I., p. 205; Varey, ed., *The Mexican Treasury: The Writings of Dr. Francisco Hernández*, p. 77.

70. Fray Bernardino de Sahagún, *Historia general de las cosas de Nueva España*, 2 vols. (México: Alianza Editorial, 1988), Vol. II, pp. 637, 641, 643, and 649; see also Carlos Viesca Teviño, "Prevención y Terapeúticas Mexicas," in *Historia general de la medicina en México*, Vol. I., ed. Alfredo López Austin and Carlos Viesca Treviño (México: UNAM, Academia Nacional de Medicina, 1984), p. 213.

71. RG, Vol. VI, p.190 and 148, Vol. V, p. 247.

72. RG, Vol. II, p. 168 and Vol. IV, p. 211; Farfán, p. 34; AMRT Miravalles, 27 de enero, 1763.

73. Bartolache, pp. 58–61.

74. Cárdenas, p. 249.

75. Thomas Gage, *Thomas Gage's Travels in the New World*, ed. with intro. J. Eric S. Thompson (Norman: University of Oklahoma Press, 1958), pp. 59–60.

76. RG, Vol. V, pp. 246–7 and Vol. II, p. 205.

77. Cárdenas, p. 293.

78. Sophie D. Coe, *America's First Cuisines* (Austin: University of Texas Press, 1994), p. 234; Jeffrey M. Pilcher, *¡Que vivan los tamales! Food and the Making of Mexican Identity* (Albuquerque: University of New Mexico Press, 1998), p. 34.

79. Sophie D. Coe and Michael D. Coe, *The True History of Chocolate* (London: Thames and Hudson, 1996), chs. 1–4.

80. Bernardino de Sahagún, *Florentine Codex: General History of the Things of New Spain*, 13 vols., ed. and trans. C. E. Dibble and A. J. O. Anderson (Salt Lake City: University of Utah Press, 1950–69, XI, pp. 154–5, XII, p. 119; Teresa L. Dillinger, et al., "Food of the Gods: Cure for Humanity? A Cultural History of the Medicinal and Ritual use of Chocolate, *Journal of Nutrition* 130 (2000), 2057S–2072S, pp. 7–9.

81. Ajofrín, Vol. I, pp. 82–3.

82. RG, Vol. II, p. 194.

83. Coe and Coe, pp. 122–3; Varey, *The Mexican Treasury*, pp. 107–9; Cárdenas, pp. 136–7; Gage, p. 157.

84. Quoted in Dillinger, et al., p. 10.

85. Farfán, p. 33–4; Bartolache, pp. 61–2; Gage, p. 158.

86. Coe and Coe, p. 28–9; Gage, p.152.

87. Cárdenas, p. 248.

88. Farfán, p. 34.

89. Margret J. Weinberger, "Pica," in *The Cambridge World History of Food*, 2 vols., eds. Kenneth F. Kiple and Kriemhild Coneè (Cambridge: Cambridge University Press, 2000), pp. 967–68, 970.

90. On European standards of feminine beauty, see Sara F. Matthews Grieco, "The Body, Appearance, and Sexuality," in *A History of Women in the West: Renaissance and Enlightenment Paradoxes*, Vol. III (Cambridge, MA: Harvard University Press, 1993), pp. 46–84; on elite portraits, see *Artes de México*, "El retrato novohispano," número 25, Julio–Agosto 1994; on casta painting, see *New World Orders: Casta Painting and Colonial Latin America* (New York: Americas Society Art Gallery, 1996).

91. Serge Gruzinski, *The Conquest of Mexico* (Cambridge, UK: Polity Press, 1993), p. 4.

92. RG, Vol. II, p. 132; PNE, p. 202.

93. Cayetano de Cabrera y Quintero, *Escudo de Armas de México* (México: Institute Mexican del Seguro Social, 1981), pp. 66–7.

94. William B. Taylor, *Drinking, Homicide, and Rebellion in Colonial Mexican Villages* (Stanford: Stanford University Press, 1979), pp. 40–1.

95. Gage, pp. 225–7.

96. PNE, p. 224.

97. Ibid., pp. 245–6.

98. Gruzinski, pp. 84–6.

99. RG, Vol. VI, p. 88.

100. PNE: pp. 189 and 161.

101. Lobera de Avila, pp. 35–6.

102. Mendez, pp. 73 and 79.

103. Georges Vigarello, *Concepts of Cleanliness: Changing attitudes in France since the Middle Ages*, trans. Jean Birrell (Cambridge: Cambridge University Press, 1988).

104. Esteyneffer, Vol. I, p. 162; Lobera de Avila, p. 25; Mendez, p. 75.

105. Farfan, p. 34; Cárdenas, p. 207.

106. Mendez, pp. 52–3, 66.

107. Mendez, p. 68; Lobera de Avila, p. 33; Farfan, p. 3.

5. ENCOUNTERING ILLNESS

One of the underlying themes in this study has been that the constant proximity of sickness and death that marked life in an age before modern medicine generated illness experiences that were very different from our own. Nowadays, most of us see our maladies as simply troublesome nuisances, exceptional intrusions into an otherwise lengthy life of good health. Only when we encounter exceptional diseases—those that are debilitating or life threatening, such as Alzheimer's disease or cancer—do they come to dominate our daily lives. Modern medicine has made such huge strides against infectious diseases, yesterday's great killers, that, at least for those of us living today in the developed world, death from typhus, smallpox, infantile diarrhea, or a bad bout of the flu is a fairly remote probability, far removed from the radar screens of our daily concerns. Not only has biomedicine increased life expectancy, making death in old age the "norm" in our conception of human life, it also has medicalized it to such an extent that the death of family members and friends usually takes place away from our view and immediate experience. Yet the ubiquity of illness and, perhaps more significantly, the shadow of death were simply part of the everyday landscape of the past. Few people's lives were untouched by the death of family members struck down in the prime of life or the loss of infants and children, circumstances most of us today would have a hard time conceiving of as common, everyday experiences. Not so for people of past centuries. The voices we have heard from in this study all testify to the ubiquity of sickness, disability, and death in New Spain. Moreover, they provide us a glimpse into a wider "sickness culture" of the period, not only the everyday beliefs about the body but also at how personal preoccupations with one's state of health interfaced with larger interpretations of social, moral and spiritual well-being, a topic that we explore later in this chapter.[1] For the moment, however, let us try to imagine the sickness culture of this lost world by considering how the high incidence of disease and deformity added to the texture of daily life.

SICKNESS CULTURE

If we had to reduce the early modern culture of sickness to one fundamental essence, surely it would be that the prevalence of so much disease caused individuals to feel a high level of anxiety on a daily basis. Rarely does any correspondence of the time fail to mention health, either the writer's own or that of family and friends. For the Condesa de Miravalles, vigilance over the state of health, that of her family and her own, was a daily obsession. Along with business and politics, health is the topic that most dominated the letters she wrote to her son-in-law, Pedro Romero de Terreros.

> . . . around here illness comes and goes. *La chica* is getting better; the doctor thinks María Antonia is suffering from *destemplanza* brought on by her *flucion* . . . she was purged, is not doing well. Joseph gave me a scare, he has been with fever for four days; and with all this I have not had time to purge myself; perhaps next week I'll do it . . .

> . . . yesterday *la chica* gave us a scare she was so sick, [although] now she is better; María Francesca is still with *reumatismo*, [poor] little angel, she has been with fever, but is now better. We must have patience in everything and give thanks to God that he looks upon us with mercy.

> . . . happy to hear María Antonia is feeling relief from sore throat and fever . . . she needs to be mindful of the weather as she is very delicate and there is much smallpox about, be careful about diet. Around here *el muchacho* that was sick is doing better, but I am a bit under the weather . . . [2]

As these letters show, early modern sufferers, along with their watchful kin, appeared to display alarm not only about serious threats to health, but about minor discomforts as well. Given contemporary beliefs about the nature of disease, everyone recognized the genuine possibility that a minor symptom could be the first sign of a major decline. This is hardly surprising in an age when resistance to infectious disease was weak and a whole host of endemic maladies—infantile diarrhea, dysentery, scarlatina, measles—very often proved fatal, above all to infants and young children. And few communities in New Spain were far enough off the beaten path to completely avoid the ravages of epidemic disease, from which so many died like flies; small wonder then that people were hypersensitive to the possibility of death at any stage in life. The letters of Spanish emigrants in sixteenth-century Mexico testify to the extensive morbidity and mortality that befell many in the New World.

> . . . of our health we inform you that we are all well, even though in this land one can never be sure of good health, as so many people presently are ill and are dying like flies . . .

> . . . and since I have come here, I have not had one day of health, because all that come to this land from Spain get a *chapetonada*, from which more than a third of them die.[3]

The usual circumstances that threatened health were magnified when people undertook a venture that was completely outside of ordinary experience such as long-distance travel by ship. We are all familiar with stories about the horrors emigrants and slaves suffered from when coming to British North America in the seventeenth and eighteenth centuries. In his work on the peopling of colonial North America, Bernard Bailyn describes, in pictographic terms, the experience of voyagers on the *Hector*, a ship that carried 189 passengers from Scotland to the north shores of Nova Scotia during the summer of 1773. If conditions on the *Hector* even came close to those of most ships crossing the Atlantic during this period, these journeys must truly have been ordeals of horror.

> The hold quickly became a pesthole. Measuring only 83 feet long, 24 feet wide, and 10 feet deep, it was lit by a few fish-oil lamps and by the light that filtered through the hatch. Such ventilation as it had also came through the hatch, and the only sanitary facilities available for the 189 passengers, almost all of whom were seasick for the first week or two, were a few wooden buckets. The voyagers were literally shelved: assigned narrow wooden straw-covered pallets stacked in tiers two feet apart . . . a few days out, disease swept through the ship—first dysentery, which debilitated, almost eviscerated, its victims and made them vulnerable to deadlier diseases; then smallpox. The chills, fevers, nausea, and erupting pustules of that deadly affliction hit the children first (71—over a third of the passengers were below the age of nine);

they lay stricken in the dark, stinking hold, their parents were helpless as they watched them suffer and fade.[4]

So many of the Spanish emigrants' letters reveal a similar experience in their crossings to the New World, forewarning prospective newcomers about the "mucho trabajo y peligro" that they will encounter on the sea. Beatriz de Carvalar and her husband Melchor Valdelomar described their nightmare voyage and its aftermath for her father in letters they wrote in the early spring of 1574. "At sea," she writes, "I suffered the most cruel sicknesses that a body could undergo." Her fellow passengers expected her to die and she made her last confession several times to a few priests who happened to be on board. Her illness continued once she disembarked in Vera Cruz and was only cured after a long convalescence and expensive medical treatment that cost "more than a good hacienda costs in this land." Back in Castile, Beatriz's father, Lorenzo Martínez de Carvalar, wants to join his daughter and her family in New Spain, but, in a separate letter, his son-in-law warns him that he must be realistic about the toll the journey will take on him and his family if they come:

> [Be advised of] the trouble and danger there is on the voyage, as it is the most you can possibly imagine, and even ignoring the dangers of the sea, the sicknesses of the land and in the ships are so great that two thirds of the people died [in our ship] and this is quite ordinary; [and] that even today Melchor and Inés still get fevers, and I have been almost finished [by this], and I am very thin and cannot return to what I was, [but] *El Señor* has worked a miracle with my wife as all the doctors of México had given up hope for her.[5]

The Valdelomar family was lucky to have survived the voyage and, as they reported in their letters, regained their health sufficiently so that they were able to buy a hacienda in Mexico City and give birth to a baby girl, "the most beautiful to be born in this land."[6]

The afflictions suffered in the Spanish *flotas* proved more costly for others, inflicting hardship long after the ships had discharged their passengers. María Díaz came to Mexico with her husband sometime during the 1570s; her story, told here in a letter to her daughter in Seville, is a common one in a time when the unexpected death of a spouse or parent could cast surviving family members into circumstances of psychological and economic insecurity. María Díaz's case is made even more poignant in that she found herself alone in a strange land:

> My daughter, this is to inform you of the great hardships and dangers that we have seen on the sea, I and your father, and certainly if I had understood the great dangers we were to know at sea, I would not have come. . . . but with all these hardships God

> was served that we should arrive safely at the port, . . . And from there we wanted to go to Mexico, but, God being served, your father became ill with diarrhea and fever, and knowing that the journey would be hard for him we waited until he was somewhat better . . . later after we arrived [in Mexico], after fifteen days he again fell sick with the same illness, and from this, God being served, he died. And I would have been, if God had been served, more content if they had buried me together with him, so as not to be a widow and abandoned so far from my natural place, and in a land where no one knows me; I would like nothing more than to return, if only there was someone who could help me. For the love of God, I beg you, daughter, that you plead with my son and your husband Pedro Díaz, that if you grant me one act of compassion, let it be this: that if it is possible, even though the road is as long and dangerous as it is, come for me . . . do not permit that I am left in this land alone and abandoned, but take me to the place where I will die among my own kind, because after salvation there is no other thing I desire more.[7]

I have quoted this letter at length because it so poignantly conveys a personal experience that must have been repeated countless times in that first century of colonialization. Perilous travel and settling in a strange land gave a new dimension to the vulnerability people already felt about their health and the consequences of death. Away from the financial and emotional support of the family—the only kind of social assistance that existed in early modern times outside of the Church—people who went to the New World put themselves at great risk, not only in terms of their health but in terms of ending up completely alone and miserable as well.

Emigrants' letters frequently relate the deaths of family members, many of them children, but young adults are often mentioned as well. Diego de Pastrana writes that within the space of five weeks he lost his two children, both of marriageable age. "And after this, there was not one thing in this life which gave us contentment, nor joy, and because of this my wife has never been happy again." Diego's wife later had two other pregnancies, both of which failed in miscarriage, "from which we are truly in a state of disconsolation, so that all that we have earned [here] gives us no joy in that God has not given us any heirs." The frequent loss of children meant that the uncertainty of inheritance was often a problem for those that had established themselves in New Spain. Antonio Farfán, who lost his son, writes his sister in Seville to bring her son to Mexico because "I do not have anyone to whom I can leave what I have." Another emigrant appeals to relatives in Pamplona that they send his nephew: "eight months ago I lost my wife to *tabardillo*, and so now I am an orphan, without wife, son or daughter."[8]

The high death rates for all ages undoubtedly heightened people's awareness to the unexpected and sudden death. In October 1593, Pedro del Castillo writes to his son about an acquaintance he had in Mexico City: "Pedro de Atienza was in this city since last Christmas, ready to leave for Castile, with twenty five thousand pesos and five unmarried daughters and one son, and God was served that during the *víspera* of San Miguel, at three in the afternoon he was good, and by nine o'clock that night he was dead."[9] This obsession with the sudden death is still evident in eighteenth-century personal correspondence as well. In her continuous contemplation on the dangers to life and limb the Condesa de Miravalles comments in a letter to her son-in-law that "from one hour to the next" one could never be sure when death would come:

> . . . God shows us this by those that have [recently] died sudden deaths; I knew a woman who a few days ago suddenly died . . . and yesterday around 12 o'clock, Don Jacinto Martines, who was visiting the house of the *leñeros*, no sooner could he say I am dying when death so suddenly grabbed him . . . and they say there was barely enough time to press his hand before the body was on its way to San Diego with great splendor and this afternoon they are burying him; and various others have died recently in childbirth, [such as] the wife of Roberto and another distant relative.[10]

Disease was matched by other dangers. Earthquakes, fires, falls from buildings and scaffolding, mishaps with tools, encounters with bandits, overturned carriages, and falls from horseback were all constant hazards, not least because without adequate emergency services, blood-loss and trauma could quickly kill. Like our highways today, the roads of New Spain were dangerous places. Emigrants' letters report many accidents with horses, that single passenger vehicle of yesterday. In 1572, Martín Fernández Cubero writes from Puebla to his nephew in Spain that he fell from his horse and broke his leg, the treatment for which cost him plenty. Bartolomé de Morales thought he would always "have to walk with crutches" after an incident on horseback left his knee dislocated: "I am thankful to God," he writes, "that they called an Indian who returned it to its rightful place, and now, blessed God, I am well."[11]

As with personal letters of the time, the painted scenes in colonial ex-votos vividly reveal the dangers of everyday life in New Spain. Outside of work accidents and natural disasters, the movement of goods and people, whether on city streets or country roads, was a frequent cause of injury or death; assault by bandits, treacherous river crossings, people caught under the wheels of carriages, and bucking horses were everyday occurrences that people who moved about feared. One seventeenth-century ex-voto dedicated to the Virgin of Zapopan reveals a well-dressed man being run over by his own carriage in the countryside. Another from the eighteenth century displays the perils people faced when crossing rivers during the summer, Mexico's wet season, as it shows a man being swept away by raging water.[12] Horses, like cars today, appear frequently in the ex-votos as a constant source of accidents. In June 1785, as José Padilla was leaving his ranch for the countryside, his horse was spooked, throwing the rider off balance so that he was dragged down the road under the horse until a stirrup finally broke, setting him free. Horses could be even more dangerous on city streets, full of people and obstacles. One ex-voto to the Virgen de la Soledad recalls in vivid detail an accident on horseback that took place late one night in the city of Oaxaca:

> On the night of Monday . . . October of 1789 Mariano Josef de Torres . . . was returning from the fiesta of the town of Tlacolula; in the street they call *las ratas* there was an open ditch dug for a pipeline; not being able to see the ditch because the night was very dark, he fell in it and found himself in great conflict because the horse fell on top of him, and fearful of the water [in the ditch], he invoked the blessed Maria la Soledad and her Christian husband Josef . . . [13]

The individuals in these accidents survived, as their ex-votos testify. But undoubtedly many others suffered the effects of serious injury in a time when emergency care was limited to the setting of bones; nothing could be done, however, for copious blood loss, ruptured organs, or severe head injury.

These brief fragments in which people recorded their encounters with sickness, injury, and death immediately reveal two things: that the maintenance of health and relief of anxiety about health were constant themes in the daily lives of premodern people; and that the high incidence of sickness did not produce a state of passiveness or fatalism toward disease. Indeed, colonial sources such as health manuals, newspapers, and personal letters reveal not only a population that was constantly monitoring its own state of health but also one that reacted vigorously against illness of any kind. The Condesa de Miravalles is a case in point. Her letters are full of health advice, remedies, recommendations about diet, bleeding and purging, managing pregnancies, and therapeutic bathing. Almost all of her letters to the Romero de Terreros family in Pachuca included medicines and instructions for their use; many of these medicines appear to be personal formulas concocted by the Condesa herself. Newspapers from the eighteenth century confirm that the continuous pursuit for efficacious remedies was of primary interest to the general public as notices and advertisements for cures abounded. *La Gaceta de México* liked to inform its readers of new remedies—available for sale by their creators, of course—for the maladies that afflicted everyone: ground scorpions to "cure *dolor de costado* in a few hours"; *pulque blanco* that "corrects" diarrhea with "great success"; Matías de Olivencia's powders for various venereal diseases; cuttings from the *Táscate* tree which "cures all classes of toothache"; and of course a "universal" cure-all which its creator claimed was an "antidote for any kind of illness."[14] We also should keep in mind, in this summary of how the concern for health textured daily life, that preventative medicine is not solely a modern phenomenon. Besides actively seeking out cures and treatments on their own, people of past centuries, like people today, paid great attention to the causes of disease and took steps to avoid it. Once again, the Condesa de Miravalle serves as an especially clear window, at least into upper-class mentality about health, with her constant prophylactic purgings and bleedings and close attention to diet.

MIRACULOUS MEDICINE

This steady search for relief from the suffering and uncertainties of sickness contains another aspect of the illness experience, one that we have not spent much time on in this study, except in terms of indigenous etiology, and that is the way in which religion shaped the encounter with disease. This topic, of course, is a critically important part of our story and, because of its many facets, really demands a more rigorous scrutiny than an exploratory study such as this one will allow. In New Spain, religion and medicine overlapped and intersected at many points, with the Catholic Church acting as one of the most important cultural agents in the evolution of Spanish American medicine. As we have seen in an earlier chapter, within the larger colonial power structure, the work of evangelization and extirpation—which, among other things, involved the scrutiny of healing techniques containing suspicious practices—worked in tandem with the Protomedicato in their attempt to forge a monopoly of university trained medical professionals and a European model of medicine. Additionally, in its pursuit to exercise Christian charity, the Church also contributed to the establishment of European patterns of medical care by building and operating hospitals all over New Spain.[15] But what if we shift our gaze downward to the individual? How was one's state of health linked to larger interpretations of moral and spiritual wellbeing? Here we approach this question with a focus on some of the ways in which religious meaning intersected with the illness experience.

Throughout much of this survey, we have been exploring lay notions about the workings of the human body—specifically how and why the body became sick, and how one was to go about keeping it well—through the prism of humoralism, that collection of concepts about health that served as a basis of Western medicine for over 1,500 years. I have argued that these concepts formed a medical framework for professional healers and lay people alike, albeit with different levels of understanding. From this viewpoint, maladies arose from physical causes, either originating outside of the individual, that is, from the natural world and thus largely beyond his or her control, or from within the body itself, for which the individual was held to be more responsible, as diet and lifestyle had direct consequences for health. Yet we must not suppose that for most people in New Spain (or, for that matter, anywhere in the early modern Western world) the origins of their bodily suffering could be wrapped up so neatly in objective laws of nature.

As Roy and Dorothy Porter note in their perceptive study of sufferers in preindustrial England: "Affliction cried out for profound answers—explanations of why this was a world of sickness at all, why innocent babes died, why pain proliferated so agonizingly, why upright, blameless, individuals were seemingly victimized by disease, no less than the feckless and the reckless."[16] These were significant questions, causing much speculation and concern, particularly in a place like colonial Mexico, where a deep native religiosity was overlaid with a strong Catholic orthodoxy on continual display in elaborate rituals. At least in the Western world, where Christianity had been a strong cultural force for centuries, sickness and sin, health and holiness had become linked in ways difficult to untangle. As one historian noted, "it is arguable that it was the experience of suffering, sickness, and death which gave birth to religious devotion in the first place; and equally, that modern medical advances (the conquest of disease, the prolongation of life) have played no small part in widespread secularization."[17]

One way to enter this complicated relationship between religion and medicine is to briefly consider how Christian theology, with its God-centered view of the world, reconciled itself with a medical tradition that explained disease in terms of natural phenomena, not divine will. The short and simple answer is: surprisingly well. Christian doctrine itself offered no exclusive theory of disease; its inclination to stress moral discipline and personal guilt easily meshed with Hippocratic notions of medicine, which viewed a person's state of health as strongly linked to his or her lifestyle, constitution, and character. Church authorities did not deny disease had natural causes, nor did physicians deny divine involvement in the laws of nature that ultimately affected human health. As one sixteenth-century physician wrote: "God put virtue in the herbs and things of the earth so that man could take care of himself and free himself from disease." General notions of disease causation were multifaceted; divine and natural causes coexisted with surprising fluidity, nurtured, no doubt, by the close link between lifestyle choices and personal morality.[18]

Pestilence, however, represented a special class of disease. Because epidemics struck so many people with the same set of symptoms at the same time, they were typically interpreted as divine punishment for collective human sins. Writing about the epidemic of 1576, the surgeon Alonso Lopez de Hinojosos concludes it was the hand of God that was ultimately responsible for this unusually severe pestilence. We can see this, he writes, because weather conditions were not extreme at this time, thus there was little "corruption of the elements" that usually lead to pestilence.[19] The priest Cayetano de Cabrera y Quintero, writing about the devastating *matlazáhuatl* epidemic that swept New Spain during the years 1736–7, refers to pestilence as a "divine war." "Sickness that comes from heaven," he writes, "also requires remedies from heaven: God is the principal and sometimes the only author of pestilence."[20] Even though the scientific discourse of the day had permeated this eighteenth-century colonial world, prompting authorities to clean up urban centers of miasma-causing material, great catastrophes such as epidemics, floods, and earthquakes were still considered signs of God's displeasure with man. The apparent contradiction in these worldviews did not make them incompatible in the real world of everyday life; rather, they formed a complementary whole, each offering a mode of explanation and practical strategies for confronting calamitous events over which people had little control. City mandates that demanded the removal of trash, offal, and deeper gravesites combined with Catholic processions, prayers, and *novenarios* to ease the acute anxiety people must have felt in the face of such devastation.

Yet Christian doctrine had evolved a complicated view of the human body, one that was to have a significant impact on the wider sickness culture evolving in New Spain. While disparaging the flesh as corrupted by sin, it also stressed the inherent sacredness contained in it as well. Like other major religions in the world, Christianity is based on a dualistic view of man, one that distinguishes between an eternal spirit or soul and the physical body, a temporal fleshy dwelling place for this soul. The human body became tainted with the brush of sin at the Fall, when man weakly surrendered to carnal lust, bringing disease, destruction, and death into the world. Yet Christian views of the body cannot be reduced to a simple disdain of the flesh; they are further complicated by the narrative of Jesus Christ, born in the flesh, and later crucified in agony on the cross. Embodiment and sacrifice are, in turn, encoded in the sacrament of the Eucharist, where the ritual ingestion of bread and wine signifies the transubstantiation of the body and blood of Christ, and thus offers the faithful hope, "not (as in many faiths) of some rather amorphous, wishy-washy life after death, but of a palpable bodily resurrection at the Last Judgment, to be followed by a heavenly resumption of physical being for the saved, and eternal hellfire torments for the dammed."[21] Christianity, then, developed a kind of double vision of corporal flesh. God punished the corrupt bodies of sinners with sickness, suffering, and sudden death, whereas the bodies and bones of saints and holy people were imbued with miracle-working properties, giving rise to a cult of healing saints throughout the European continent and later the Hispanic

New World. This quest for miracle cures became an integral part of the cultural landscape in both colonial and modern Mexico.

In his classic study of medieval and early modern belief systems in England, Keith Thomas makes the following observation about why people turn to religion in the first place:

> Nearly every primitive religion is regarded by its adherents as a medium for obtaining supernatural power. This does not prevent it from functioning as a system of explanation, a source of moral injunctions, a symbol of social order, or a route to immorality; but it does mean that it also offers the prospect of a supernatural means of control over man's earthly environment. The history of early Christianity offers no exception to this rule. Conversions to the new religion, whether in the time of the primitive Church or under the auspices of the missionaries of more recent times, have frequently been assisted by the belief of converts that they are acquiring not just a means of other-worldly salvation, but a new and more powerful magic.

Although the Catholic Church itself did not claim to work miracles, it derived enormous prestige from those of its members who seemed to possess a special access to God.[22] The Spanish creation of New Spain—that grandiose amalgam of colonialization and evangelization—certainly benefited from the proliferation of divine images with miraculous powers that quickly sprang up throughout the Mexican countryside, a process greatly aided by existing Mesoamerican patterns of religiosity. As we have seen in our examination of indigenous notions of the body, one's state of health was directly linked to the demands and whims of the various gods. Mesoamerican religion exhibited striking similarities with popular Spanish Catholicism, which centered on local images of saints with specialized supernatural powers. In early modern Spain, the religious devotion of common people was very localized: universal figures including Mary and Christ became particularized to specific places; thus, Our Lady of Riansares or the Christ of Urda, became valued for local believers above other Marys and Christs.[23] In his extensive study of Nahua life after the conquest, James Lockhart notes that indigenous Catholicism was mostly about saints. "No other aspect of Christian religious belief and ritual had a remotely comparable impact on the broad range of their activity (especially if we consider that Jesus Christ and often the cross were in effect treated as so many more saints)." By the seventeenth century, most indigenous households possessed one or more images of saints. Although Church doctrine repeatedly emphasized the distinction between representation and the entity being represented, the Nahuas (and much of the Spanish population as well) continued to view the spiritual being and the tangible form as fully integrated. "What the Nahuas had in their houses *were* the saints, in a particular manifestation, and they constantly spoke of them correspondingly."[24] By the end of the first century of Spanish rule, the accumulated anecdotal evidence of miracles had given rise to a network of shrines throughout much of the colony. Different saints appealed to different groups and regions, and many of these intercessors were known for their specialties. The Virgen de los Remedios, for example, protected against drought, that of Guadalupe against floods, the Virgen de los Dolores assisted maidens and widows in danger of losing their honor, San Ignacio de Loyola helped women in labor, San Lázaro was called on by those suffering from diseases of the skin, and San José offered help in earthquakes.[25]

The miracles associated with these saints clearly conformed to the normal operation of both the Spanish and indigenous worlds; *novohispanos* in the grip of affliction felt that divine help was an option to them, particularly when "earthly" help had failed to produce results. Given the efficacy of contemporary medicine to prevent and cure the devastating diseases of the time, it is no surprise that healing saints stood firmly alongside domestic remedies and local medical practitioners in the marketplace for relief.

Just how much significance did people give to divine intervention in human health? From our thoroughly secularized point of view, a glance back to the people of earlier centuries reveals, on the surface at least, an almost fatalistic sensibility about the power of God over human well-being. Clearly, both the Spanish and Mesoamerican populations of New Spain possessed cultures that encouraged them to fear the consequences of their personal (and collective) behavior. But, as I have argued throughout this book, colonial Mexicans were anything but fatalistic about being sick; religion had no monopoly in explaining illness, although it certainly entered into the layers of causes. Nor indeed is this a question that can be answered with broad generalizations: individuals were different, as were the circumstances of their ailments. Emigrants' letters from the sixteenth century never mention health without mentioning God's will—death, illness, and good health all come to pass because God is thus served—although the modern reader senses a formulaic quality already forming here. Only one letter writer offers an interpretation of why he spent fifty-two days sick in bed: "it was a punishment for some sins and a correction of those to come." he writes to his wife back home in Seville.[26] By contrast, God's will is rarely mentioned two hundred years later in the letters of the Condesa de Miravalle. This is not to say that she does not believe that divine intervention is at work around her; she clearly does, as is evident in the visits she and her daughter pay to various shrines in Mexico City in order to pray for the health of family members. But her view of medicine and religion is that of a more equitable partnership: "although all of us are subject to the will of God," she writes to her son-in-law, "we still need to put forth our part in everything."[27]

Some of the most vivid examples of the linkage between spirituality and sickness are manifested in the ex-votos of the period. The Latin word *ex-voto* means "of a vow" and it designates an object offered to God, the Virgin, or the saints as a response to a favor received. These votive offerings are different from other types of offerings left at shrines and chapels, such as candles, gifts of food, or monetary offerings, in that they always indicate a close relationship to the person and/or event from which the vow originated. Taking diverse forms, they are often personal objects that speak to the miracle at hand such as clothing, eyeglasses, photographs, and letters, or items bought expressly for the shrine like miniature tin limbs or hearts. The ex-votos—or, as they are sometimes called in Mexico, *retablos*—referred to in this study are even more unique: painted scenes, usually accompanied by text, both of which refer to the portentous event that motivated it. The texts are often expressed in commemorative language such as "with this *retablo* I offer thanks" and usually give various details about the beneficiary and situation.[28] These votive offerings are created specifically to be put on display in the shrines of a particular virgin, saint, or Christ figure to publicize their supernatural powers, a process that promotes the reputation of the divine image and, in turn, that of the shrine and its keepers as well. In essence, then, the ex-voto is a promise materialized into an object, the likes of which represents a reciprocal and successfully executed transaction between an individual and a divine image. In Mexico, votive painting became most firmly established among the popular mestizo classes during the nineteenth century, although it first emerged as a creole practice during the early colonial era.[29]

Certainly, the most impressive characteristic of ex-votos is the desperation of the supplicant. A word often used in the descriptive text is *desahuiciado*, to be completely without hope. The ones that depict situations of illness and disability are graphic snapshots of people who have exhausted all "earthly" efforts; the medicines, the bleedings, and the purgings have not helped; thus, the only prospect left is a miracle. Doña Maria Flores, an upper class woman of the late eighteenth century, finds herself with a "grave apoplexy of blood, without any hope of remedy" Her invocation to the Virgin of Guadalupe—by this time the foremost divine image in all of Mexico—is granted and she is left "good and healthy." The gravity of the sufferers' condition is conveyed not only by the painted scenes, but often by the language used to describe the effects of the illness itself, a language that can be quite melodramatic. Words like, "cruel and mortal," "agony," "anguish," and "torment," are used to great effect in conveying the visceral quality of suffering. Another eighteenth-century ex-voto, this time that of a priest at a convent in the town of Pazcuaro, is suffering from "*un mal de orina* so cruel and mortal," caused by a kidney stone that he fears will kill him. As anyone who has passed a stone through the urinary tract will attest, the intensity of pain is excruciating. As he lies there, "in *agonia*, with little hope of life and being in this state of anguish," the image of Nuestra Señora de la Salud is brought into the bedroom by other priests of the convent. And "at that very instant he passed the stone, the affliction was over and life was granted."[30] As in so many of the ex-votos, the there can be no doubt that the sufferer's recovery was of a miraculous nature. Patients do not gradually get better as they would if being treated by a physician; rather, recovery is sudden and unequivocal.

This amalgam of religion and medicine is not limited to the asking for favors from celestial images but also can be found physically in the natural elements at many of the shrines. One four-part ex-voto displays four miraculous cures attributed to the archangel San Miguel, a popular saint with both the creole and Indian communities in New Spain. In each one of these cures, the sufferers are healed either by drinking the water from the shrine, presumably either well water or a stream running through the holy site, or by having soil rubbed onto their skin. "They carried Sebastian Hernandez to the sanctuary, desperate [*desahuiciado*] and very swollen with dropsy, and rubbing him with dirt he was cured after three days." Another sufferer is "*desahuiciado* with *lamparones y empeines*," severe skin afflictions, but he, too, is cured after the holy soil is rubbed on him, as is another man who is suffering from "one hundred and ten sores." And lastly, a whole town of Indians is cured of "*un gran peste*" by drinking the water of the shrine and having "the holy soil" applied to their bodies.

The promise to perform the vow—that is, to produce the ex-voto, make a pilgrimage to the image's shrine, and display the evidence of the miracle—appears to have been a serious matter. Failure to do so could provoke castigating action from the offended saint, resulting in a relapse of the illness, or worse, a more serious affliction than the original one. The ex-voto of little Hipólito poignantly reveals this aspect of the negotiation process between mortals and miracle-workers. The supplicants in this case are the worried parents of the five-month old Hipólito (who, in the painting, looks more like a miniature adult than a baby). The child is quite sick, although the text does not give us much information about the nature of his illness, only that he has "two *postemas* under his arms," and that he was placed in some sort of binding for two days which made it impossible for him to move. His parents, "Don Manuel Varrios and Doña Catarina Ximenes Colon, Spaniards [and] residents of this city," promise to commission a *lienzo*, or painting, of the suffering child for the Virgen de la Soledad, the patron saint of the city of Oaxaca, and hang it in her shrine if he is cured of his malady. Although much of the text is illegible, it is possible to piece together what happened next. The child does get better, in fact, at one point, he is "perfectly well"; but the parents, by "having delayed in preparing the painting," unwittingly brought more bad health to their son. The child now starts to show bizarre symptoms: "not being able to move his feet, or his hands, everything completely twisted, and after this, many other *accidentes* befell him, all of them *mortales*, until the realization came that everything was on account of not carrying out the promise [made to the Virgin]."[31] The failure of Hipólito's parents to carry out their vow in a timely fashion was met, in their minds at least, with clear retribution: the recurrence of their son's illness. As for poor Hipólito, we can not know from this ex-voto if he ultimately survived these childhood illnesses or not. With infant mortality rates still somewhere near 30 percent, there is a high probability that he ended up like so many of his contemporaries, dead in the first year of life.

Apparently, the failure to carry out a vow could produce weighty consequences for a life time. Another very interesting ex-voto to come out of eighteenth-century Mexico relates an elaborate tale of a broken vow that affects a family's health through several decades. The original promise is given to San Miguel by Don Antonio de Veray and Doña Catalina Orits during the birth of their daughter, who was born prematurely and, according to the parents, would have died had it not been for the miracle-working powers of the archangel. Unfortunately, Don Antonio and his wife were quite lax about keeping their end of the bargain and did not follow through with placing a painting in San Miguel's sanctuary. Then, as the daughter reached the age of *doncella*, or late adolescence, she began to experience strange and severe afflictions: "blood came out of her mouth and eyes, with *mortales agonias*, she suffered for five years and each day her symptoms were worse, and from this she developed interior sores [*llagas interiores*] in her back, so that she could neither be in bed, sitting, or standing because it penetrated to her bones, nerves, and entrails, [so much that] she was just waiting to die." The young lady's parents now became aware of their awful mistake. "Now the demand from San Miguel had arrived and [Don Antonio] promised him to have the *milagro* painted . . . if this time he would cure her." Once again, the saint was generous with his miraculous powers and in nineteen days she was cured without any remedy other than having the image [*estampa*] of San Miguel placed on her back." Remarkably, again the parents posponed completing their vow for another year and a half, in which time the daughter's symptoms returned. Ultimately, however, San Miguel was charitable to this family once the vow was carried out; not only did the *doncella* recover, but the saint eventually cured two brothers of Don Antonio, both of which were "gravely and incurably ill," and another daughter, "on the verge of death from bloody dysentery," as well. Favorite saints and virgins were thus genuine players in the marketplace for cures, but this was by no means a one-way transaction. The supplicant's failure to keep his or her end of the bargain, that is, to publicize the miracle, thereby boosting the reputation of the saint, carried potential consequences.

The illness experiences that come to us through these ex-votes underscore what has been a constant theme in this study: that the combination of widespread illness, particularly infectious diseases, and the inadequacies of contemporary medicine meant that all social groups in colonial Mexico directed a great deal of attention to health in everyday life. We have seen how this search for relief from sickness generated a very broad spectrum of practitioners promoting an equally diverse array of healing strategies, most of them combining both rational and supernatural practices in varying degrees. The ex-votos examined here clearly mark the final point in the "hierarchy of resort," for those that were *desahuiciado*, without any hope of human remedy.

BY WAY OF CONCLUSION

The central purpose of this investigation has been to explore the beliefs ordinary people in Mexico's past had about health and illness. Beginning with a seemingly simple question—How did people explain why they fell sick?—this study has attempted to map out the basic notions—both Spanish and indigenous—about human health that circulated during Mexico's colonial years. Because these frameworks are deeply embedded in how people view the relationship between their own physicality and the material conditions in which they live, they bring to light those aspects of everyday life that are most commonly shared: the impact of personal lifestyle, climate, and supernatural intervention on the well-being of individuals. How these diverse belief systems clashed and evolved in New Spain promises to be a fertile ground for future investigations.

Several potential research topics emerged from this survey—that is, the role medical practitioners, both legally sanctioned and not, played in the complex dynamics between ideology and the actual practice of colonial rule; the ways in which ideas about gender shaped the practice of medicine; the *mestizaje* of popular medical beliefs, both indigenous and European, the remnants of which are still visible in Mexican folk medicine today—but none of them was pursued in any depth. Instead, I have centered my focus on the frameworks that laypeople used to make sense of health. To do this, I have tried to get as close as possible to the everyday world of colonial Mexico, where we would expect common notions about health to be most visible, by exploring the diseases and ailments people claimed to suffer from, the medical market place in which they sought relief, the conceptions people had about the inner workings of the body, and divine influence on human health.

Because of its cultural diversity colonial Mexico makes an especially rich setting to explore premodern concepts of health and disease. As one of only two areas of high civilization in the Americas before 1492, Mesoamerica was home to various peoples with a long tradition of empiric and shamanistic medicine. Prehispanic doctors combined sophisticated hands-on skills, especially in the fields of wound treatment, obstetrics, and herbal remedies with elaborate rituals linking them to a supernatural world that exerted a great deal of influence over human health. Indigenous etiology was firmly rooted in basic assumptions about how the world was structured. Human beings lived at the center of a universe in which cosmic forces affected all aspects of human life. In contrast to a Christian cosmology that viewed nature as a passive creation, the Mesoamerican universe was a very animate place; all features of the physical world—the mountains, the wind, bodies of water, the sun, and the sky—were active forces associated with various deities. Many deities were represented as male-female pairs, or as embodiments of contrasting characteristics such as fertility and death, or creation and destruction, reflecting the dualism that underlay much of native culture. Destructive, chaotic forces were as necessary to life as were the creative, positive forces, each depending on the other for its functioning.

The challenge for humans then was to constantly strive for a proper equilibrium, the right balance between order and chaos. As we have seen, illness was strongly associated with a tip to the disorder side of things. Any immoderation or excess—over indulgence in food, drink, or sex—or any exposure to "filth" in both a physical or moral sense could make one ill. Mirroring the physical world around them, Mesoamerican bodies contained several animate forces—the *teyolia*, *ihiyotl*, and *tonalli*—that were responsible for vital bodily functions in tangible ways, such as body temperature, growth, and breathing. Yet they also appear to have been the means through which supernatural powers, usually triggered by immoderate human behavior, manifested themselves inside the body.

In the sixteenth century, conquering Spaniards began to superimpose a European worldview on this indigenous world—insisting on Spanish forms of settlement and local government, spreading the tenets of Christianity, imposing European notions of race and class, and forever changing native patterns of production and consumption. A European etiology, based on the ancient texts of Hippocrates and Galen, was an essential part of this imported worldview. Classically trained professionals and laypeople alike offered similar explanations for why people fell sick: the body's four humors had been thrown out of balance, causing one or more of these fluids to be in disequilibrium with the others. An imbalance's origins could be found in an endless combination of factors; depending on one's stage of life and individual temperament, exposure to all sorts of environmental phenomena—north winds, cold rain, heavy mists, miasma-laden air—could bring on ill health. The influence of lifestyle was equally significant, as eating the wrong foods, too much or too little exercise, and sexual intercourse at the wrong time could upset the delicate balance that was health. These ideas coexisted, sometimes quite comfortably, with widely held beliefs that sickness also could be the result of divine will or a more earthly bound form of supernaturalism, that of witchcraft and magic.

How did these Spanish and Mesoamerican notions about the body evolve in a colonial milieu where the degree of contact between the two cultures was a driving force in change? In more isolated indigenous communities, the few extant sources to shed any light on colonial indigenous medicine suggest that preconquest beliefs and practices survived virtually intact well into the seventeenth century.[32] With time, as the Spanish Mexican world pushed ever farther into the countryside, such overtly preconquest practices must have either receded accordingly or become overlaid with European, and especially Christian, elements. Certainly these two worldviews, and their corresponding beliefs about managing sickness and health, became more entangled as the mestizo population grew in the late seventeenth and eighteenth centuries, although this blending was by no means symmetrical. The fusion of indigenous and European medical approaches was also undoubtedly aided by the apparent similarities both systems shared. Both defined health as a state of equilibrium, a balance that needed constant maintenance, and both charted vital changes in that equilibrium through a mapping of hot and cold qualities. Both systems had similar ideas about "ridding" the body of its disturbance, forcing the illness "out" through a variety of methods that purged, either via the stomach, intestines, or urinary track. And, finally, both systems were highly holistic, emphasizing the influence of physical as well as mental conditions on overall health. In this sense, then, the humoral medicine brought by the Spanish in the sixteenth century provided a logical and simple framework on which indigenous—and, later, mestizo—popular curing practices could be hung.

NOTES

1. For more on "sickness culture," see Roy Porter, *Disease, Medicine and Society in England, 1550–1860* (Cambridge: Cambridge University Press, 1993), pp. 17–18.

2. AMRT, *Miravalles*, 21 de julio, 1757, 13 de julio 1759, 12 de noviembre, 1761.

3. "Juan de León, Leonor de Espinosa y Juan Hipólito de Espinosa al padre de ella Alvaro de Espinosa, en Alcalá de Henares," Puebla: 31 de marzo, 1566; "Alonso de Alocer a su hermano Juan de Colonia, en Madrid," México: 10 de deciembre, 1577, in Enrique Otte, *Cartas privadas de emigrantes a Indias, 1540–1616* (México: Fondo de Cultura Económica, 1996), pp. 149–50, 98–9.

4. Bernard Bailyn, *Voyagers to the West: A Passage in the Peopling of America on the Eve of the Revolution* (New York: Vintage Books, 1986), p. 394.

5. "Beatriz de Carvallar a su padre Lorenzo Martínez de Carvallar, en Fuentes de León," México: 10 de marzo, 1574, and "Melchor Valdelomar a su suegro Lorenzo Martínez de Carvallar, en Fuentes de León, Veracruz: 22 de marzo, 1574, in Otte, pp. 84–6.

6. Ibid., p. 85.

7. "María Díaz a su hija Inés Díaz, en Sevilla," México: 31 de marzo, 1577, ibid., pp. 97–8.

8. "Diego de Pastrana a su tío Juan Díaz, en Fuentelaencia," Puebla: 30 de abril, 1571; "Antonio Farfán a su hermana Catalina Farfán, en Sevilla," México: 4 de abril, 1576; "Alonso Martinez de la Cunza y Arbizu a su hermano Juan Martinez de la Cunza y Arbizu, en Pamplona," México: 15 de augosto, 1589, Otte, pp. 153, 95, 117.

9. "Pedro del Castillo a su hijo Pedro de Castillo en Torija," México: 1 de octubre, 1593, in Otte, p. 126.

10. AMRT, *Miravalles*, 28 de julio, 1757.

11. "Martín Fernández Cubero a su sobrino Pedro Hernández Cubero, en Fuentelaencina," Puebla: 21 de marzo, 1572, in Otte, pp. 154–55; "Bartolomé de Morales a su padre Antón Pérez, en Sevilla," México: 30 de octubre, 1573, in Otte, pp. 72–3.

12. River crossing: ex-voto de Manuel Sanchez, July 1777, Museo de la Soledad, Oaxaca, Mexico.

13. Ex-voto de Mariano Josef de Torres, Museo de la Soledad, Oaxaca, Mexico.

14. *Gaceta de México*, "Sultepec," marzo de 1729, Vol. III, n. 16, p. 127; "México," mayo de 1737, Vol. I, n. 114, p. 910; "Encargos," martes 12 de julio de 1792, Vol. IV, n. 37, p. 352; "Sand Luis Potosí, 9 de febrero," martes 23 de marzo de 1790, Vol. IV, n. 6, p. 43; "México," diciembre de 1732, Vol. I, n. 61, pp. 484–5.

15. For more on the Church's involvement in medicine, see Francisco Guerra, "The Role of Religion in Spanish American Medicine," in *Medicine and Culture*, ed. F. N. L. Poynter (London: Wellcome Institute of the History of Medicine, 1969).

16. Roy Porter and Dorothy Porter, *In Sickness and in Health: The British Experience, 1650–1850* (London: Fourth Estate, 1988), p. 166.

17. Roy Porter, "Religion and Medicine," in CEHM, Vol. II, p. 1449.

18. Ibid., p. 1452; Juan de Cárdenas, *Problemas y secretos maravillosos de las Indias*, intro. and notes by Angeles Durán (Madrid: Alianza Editorial, 1988), p. 268.

19. Alonoso López de Hinojosos. *Suma y recopilación de cirugía con un arte para sangrar muy uútil y provechosa* (México: Academia Nacional de Medicina, 1977), p. 210.

20. Cayetano de Cabrera y Quintero, *Escudo de Armas de México* (México: Instituto Mexicano del Seguro Social, 1981), p. 25.

21. Roy Porter, "Religion and Medicine," in CEHM, Vol. II, pp. 1450–1.

22. Keith Thomas, *Religion and the Decline of Magic* (New York: Charles Scribner's Sons, 1971), p. 25–6.

23. William A. Christian Jr., *Local Religion in Sixteenth-Century Spain* (Princeton, NJ: Princeton University Press, 1981), p. 178.

24. James Lockhart, *The Nahuas after the Conquest: A Social and Cultural History of the Indians of Central Mexico, Sixteenth through Eighteenth Centuries* (Stanford: Stanford University Press, 1992), pp. 235–8.

25. Pilar Gonzalbo Aizpuru, "Lo prodigioso cotidiano en los exvotos novohispanos," in *Dones y promesas: 500 años de arte ofrenda (exvotos mexicanos)* (México D.F: Fundación Cultural Televisa, A.C. and Centro Cultural/Arte Contemporáneo A.C., 1996), p. 51.

26. "Hernán Ruiz a su mujer Mariana de Montedoca, en Sevilla," México: 21 de octubre, 1584, in Otte, p. 108.

27. AMRT, *Miravalles*, 24 de marzo, 1757, 9 de agosto, 1762, 31 de agosto 1759.

28. María del Carmen Medina San Román, "Votive Art: Miracles of Two Thousand Years," in *Folk Art of Spain and the Americas: El Alma del Pueblo*, ed. Marion Oettinger Jr. (San Antonio, TX: San Antonio Museum of Art, 1997), p. 109.

29. Jorge Durand and Douglas S. Massey, *Miracles on the Border: Retablos of Mexican Migrants to the United States* (Tucson: University of Arizona Press, 1995), pp. 12–13; Gloria Fraser Giffords, *Mexican Folk Retablos*, rev. ed. (Albuquerque: University of New Mexico Press, 1994), 143–4.

30. Ibid. (cat. 98), p. 51.

31. Ex-voto de Hipólito, 1743, Museo de la Soledad, Oaxaca, Mexico.

32. Hernando Ruiz de Alarcón, *Treatise on the Heathen Superstitions that Today Live among the Indians Native to this New Spain*, 1629, trans. and ed. J. Richard Andrews and Ross Hassig (Norman: University of Oklahoma Press, 1984).

ABBREVIATIONS

Works frequently cited have been identified by the following abbreviations:

AMRT	*Archivo Manuel Romero de Terreros*
CEHM	*Companion Encyclopedia of the History of Medicine.* Edited by W.F. Bynum and Roy Porter. 2 volumes. London: Routledge, 1993.
PNE	*Papeles de Nueva España publicados de orden y con fondos del gobierno mexicano por Francisco del Paso y Troncoso.* 2a serie, *Geográfica y Estadística*, México: Editoral Cosmos, 1979.
RG	*Relaciones Geográficas del siglo XVI.* Edited by René Acuña. 6 volumes. México: Universidad Nacional Autónoma de México, 1982–85.

BIBLIOGRAPHY

Aguirre Beltran, Gonzalo. 1963 *Medicina y magia: el proceso de aculturación en la estructura colonial*. México: Institutio Nacional Indigenista.

Ajofrín, P. Fray Francisco de. 1958 *Diario del viaje que por orden de la sagrada congregación de propaganda fide hizo a la América septentrional en el siglo XVIII el P. Fray Francisco Ajofrín Capuchino*. Madrid: Archivo Documental Español.

Anzures y Bolaños, Ma. de Carmen. 1983 *La medicina tradicional en México: proceso histórico, sincretismos y conflictos*. México: Universidad Nacional Autónoma de México.

Arias de Benavides, Pedro. 1992 *Secretos de Cirugía*. Edited by Juan Somolinos Palencia. México: Academia Nacional de Medicina.

Arrizabalaga, Jon, John Henderson, and Roger French. 1997 *The Great Pox: The French Disease in Renaissance Europe*. New Haven: Yale University Press.

The Badianus Manuscript. 1940 Introduction, translation, and annotations by Emily Walcott Emmart. Baltimore: The Johns Hopkins Press.

Bakewell, Peter. 1997 *A History of Latin America: Empires and Sequels, 1450–1930*. Oxford: Blackwell Publishers.

Bartolache, José Ignacio. 1983 *Mercurio Volante (1772–1773)*. México: Universidad Nacional Autónoma de México.

Bauer, Arnold J. 1990 "Millers and Grinders: Technology and Household Economy in Meso-America." *Agricultural History* 64, no.1 (Winter): 1–17.

——. 2001 *Goods, Power, History: Latin America's Material Culture*. Cambridge: Cambridge University Press.

Bélard, Maríanne & Philippe Verrier. 1996 *Los exvtotos del occidente de México*. México: El Colegio de Michoacán y Centre Français D'Études Mexicaines et Centraméricaines.

Bonfil Batalla, Guillermo. 1996 *Mexico Profundo: Reclaiming a Civilization*. Translated by Philip A. Dennis. Austin: University of Texas Press.

Brandt, Allan M. 1993 "Sexually Transmitted Diseases." In *Companion Encyclopedia of the History of Medicine*, vol. 1.Edited by W.F. Bynum and Roy Porter. London: Routledge.

Bustamante, Miguel E. 1982 "La fiebre amarilla en México y su origen en América." In *Ensayos sobre la historia de las epidemias en México*. Edited by Enrique Florescano and Elsa Malvido Miranda. México: Instituto Mexicano del Seguro Social.

Cabrera y Quintero, Cayetano. 1981 *Escudo de Armas de Mexcio. Escrito por el presbítero Cayetano de Cabrera y Quintero para conmemorar el final de la funesta epidemia de matlazáhuatl que asoló a la Nueva España entre 1736 y 1738*. Edición facsimilar con un estudio histórico y una cronología de Victor M. Ruiz Naufal. México: Instituto Mexicano de Seguro Social.

Calderon de la Barca, Fanny. 1946 *Life in Mexico, During a Residence of Two Years in that Country*. New York: E.P.Dutton and Company.

Cárdenas, Juan de. 1988 *Problemas y secretos maravillosos de las Indias*. Madrid: Alianza Editorial.

Cárdenas de la Peña, Enrique, editor. 1992 *Temas medicos de la Nueva*. México: Instituto Cultural Domecq, A.C.

Cartas de Indias. 1877 Madrid.

Cervantes de Salazar, Francisco. 1972 *México en 1554 y Túmulo imperial*. Edited by Edmundo O'Gorman. México: Editorial Porrúa.

Christian, William A. Jr. 1981 *Local Religion in Sixteenth-Century Spain*. Princeton: Princeton University Press.

——. 1989 *Person and God in a Spanish Village*. Rev. ed. Princeton: Princeton University Press.

——. 1991 "Secular and Religious Responses to a Child's Potentially Fatal Illness." In *Religious Regimes and State Formation: Perspectives from European Ethnology*. Edited by Eric Wolf. Albany: State University of New York Press.

Ciudad Real, Antonio de. 1993 *Tratado curioso y docto de las grandezas de la Nueva España*. 2 Vols. Edited by Josefina García Quintana and Víctor M. Castillo Farreras. México: Universidad Nacional Autónoma de México.

Clouse, Michelle Lee. 2004 "Administering and Administrating Medicine: Regulation of the Medical Marketplace in Philip II's Spain," Ph.D. diss., University of California, Davis.

Cockburn, Aiden T. 1971 "Infectious Disease in Ancient Populations," *Current Anthropology*, 12, pp. 45–66.

Coe, Sophie D. 1994 *America's First Cuisines*. Austin: University of Texas Press.

Coe, Sophie D. and Michael D. Coe. 1996 *The True History of Chocolate*. London: Thames and Hudson.

Cohen, Mark Nathan. 1989 *Health and the Rise of Civilization.* New Haven: Yale University Press.

Cook, Harold J. 1993 "Physical Methods." In *Companion Enclyclopedia of the History of Medicine,* vol. 2. Edited by W.F. Bynum and Roy Porter. London: Routledge.

Cook, Noble David. 1998 *Born to Die: Disease and New World Conquest, 1492–1650.* Cambridge: Cambridge University Press.

Cook, Noble David and W.George Lovell. 1991 "Unraveling the Web of Disease," in *Secret Judgements of God: Old World Disease in Colonial Spanish America.* Edited by Noble David Cook and W.Geogre Lovell. Norman: Univeristy of Oklahoma Press.

Cook, Shelburne. 1937 *The Extent and Significance of Disease Among the Indians of Baja California, 1697–1813.* Berkeley: University of California.

——. 1940 "The Smallpox Epidemic of 1797 in Mexico." *Bulletin of the History of Medicine,* VII, pp.937–969.

——. 1946 "The Incidence and Significance of Disease Among the Aztecs and Related Tribes." *The Hispanic American Historical Review,* vol. 26, pp.320–35.

Cook, Shelburne F. and Woodrow Borah. 1971–9 *Essays in Population History.* 3 vols. Berkeley: University of California Press.

Cooper, Donald B. 1965 *Epidemic Disease in Mexico City 1761–1831: An Administrative, Social, and Medical Study.* Austin: University of Texas Press.

Corbin, Alain. 1986 *The Foul and the Fragrant: Odor and the French Social Imagination.* Leamington Spa: Berg Publishers.

Crosby, Alfred W. 1972 *The Columbian Exchange: Biological Consequences of 1492.* Westport: Greenwood Press.

——. 1986 *Ecological Imperialism: the Biological Expansion of Europe, 900–1900.* Cambridge: Cambridge University Press.

Cueny Mateo, Miguel Ángel. 1999 *Puebla de los Ángeles en los tiempos de una peste colonial: una mirada en torno al matlazahuatl de 1737.* Zamora, Mich.: El Colegio de Michoacán, Benemérita Universidad Autónoma de Puebla.

De Vos, Paula. 2001 "The Art of Pharmacy in Seventeenth- and Eighteenth-Century Mexico." Ph.D. diss., University of California, Berkeley.

Diamond, Jared. 1999 *Guns, Germs, and Steel: the Fates of Human Societies.* New York: W.W. Norton & Company.

Díaz del Castillo, Bernal. 1991 *Historia verdadera de la conquista de la Nueva España.* México: Alianza Editorial.

Dillinger, Teresa L. et al. 2000 "Food of the Gods: Cure for Humanity? A Cultural History of the Medicinal and Ritual use of Chocolate." *Journal of Nutrition,* http://jn.nutrition.org/cgi/content/full/130/8/2057S.

Dobyns, Henry F. 1993 "Disease Transfer at Contact." *Annual Review of Anthropolgy,* Vol. 22, 1993, pp. 273–91.

Dones y promesas: 500 años de arte ofrenda (exvotos mexicanos). 1996 Mexico, D.F: Fundación Cultural Televisa, A.C. and Centro Cultural/Arte Contemporáneo. A.C.

Durand, Jorge & Douglas S. Massey. 1995 *Miracles on the Border: Retablos of Mexican Migrants to the United States.* Tucson: University of Arizona Press.

Emch-Dériaz, Antoinette. 1990 "The Non-naturals Made Easy, in *The Popularization of Medicine, 1650–1850*. Edited by Roy Porter. London: Routledge.

Epistolario de Nueva España, 1505–1818. 1940 Francisco del Paso y Troncoso, editor. 16 vols. México: Biblioteca Historica Mexicana de Obras Ineditas.

Esquivel Otea, Ma. Teresa, 1977 *Indice de los ramos hospitales y Protomedicato*. México: Archivo General de la Nacion.

Esteyneffer, Juan de. 1978 *Florilegio Medicinal de todas las enfermedades sacado de varios y clásicos autores para bien de los pobres y de los que tienen falta de médicos*. 2 vols. Edited by Ma. del Carmen Anzures y Bolaños. México: Academia Nacional de Medicina.

Fajardo Ortiz, Guillermo. 1980 *Breve historia de los hospitales de la Ciudad de México*. México: Asociación Mexicana de Hospitales, A.C./Sociedad Mexicana de Historia y Filosofía de la Medicina.

Farfán, Augustín, 1944 *Tractado breve de medicina y de todas las enfermedades*. Madrid: Ediciones Cultura Hispanica.

Feliciano, Zaida M. 2000 "Mexico's Demographic Transformation: 1920 to 1900." In *A Population History of North America*. Edited by Michael R. Haines and Richard H.Steckel. Cambridge: Cambridge University Press.

Fernández del Castillo, Francisco. 1936 *La cirugia mexicana en los siglos XVI & XVII*. New York: E.R. Squibb & Sons.

——. 1953 *La Facultad de Medicina segun el archivo de la Real y Pontifica Universidad de Mecidina*. México: Consejo de Humanidades.

Fernández de Castillo, Francisco and Alicia Hernández Torres. 1965 *El Tribunal del Protomedicato en la Nueva España, segun el archivo hístorico de la Facultad de Medicina*. México: Universidad Nacional Autónoma de México.

Florescano, Enrique and Elsa Malvido Miranda, editors. 1982 *Ensayos sobre la historia de las epidemias en México*. 2 vols. México: Instituto Mexicano del Seguro Social.

Foster, George M. 1992 *Hippocrates' Latin American Legacy: Humoral Medicine in the New World*. Amsterdam: Gordon and Breach Science Publishers.

La Gaceta de México. Mexico City.

Gage, Thomas. 1958 *Thomas Gage's Travels in the New World*. Edited by J. Eric S. Thompson. Norman: University of Oaklahoma Press.

García Acosta, Virginia, editor. 1992 *Estudios históricos sobre desastres naturales en México: balance y perspectivas*, México: Centro de Investigaciones y Estudios Superiores en Antropología Social.

García Icazbalceta, Joaquín, editor. 1866 *Colección de documentos para la historia de México*. México.

——. 1954 *Bibliografía mexicana del Siglo XVI*. México: Fondo de Cultura Económica.

Gerhard, Peter. 1993 *A Guide to the Historical Geography of New Spain*. Rev. ed. Norman: University of Oklahoma Press.

Gibson, Charles. 1964 *The Aztecs Under Spanish Rule: A History of the Indians of the Valley of Mexico, 1519–1810*. Stanford: Stanford University Press.

Giffords, Gloria Fraser. 1992 *Mexican Folk Retablos*. Rev. ed. Albuquerque: University of New Mexico Press.

Granjel, Luis S. 1978–1981 *Historia General de la Medicina Española*. 5 vols. Salamanca: Ediciones Universidad de Salamanca.

Granshaw, Lindsay. 1993 "The Hospital." In *Companion Encyclopedia of the History of Medicine*, vol. 2. Edited by W.F. Bynum and Roy Porter. London: Routledge.

Griffith, James S. 1992 *Beliefs and Holy Places: A Spiritual Geography of the Primeria Alta*. Tucson: University of Arizona Press.

Gruzinski, Serge. 1996 *Painting the Conquest: The Mexican Indians and the European Renaissance*. Translated by Deke Dusinberre. Paris: Unesco/Flammarion.

——. 1993 *The Conquest of Mexico: The Incorporation of Indian Societies into the Western World, 16th–18th Centuries*. Translated by Eileen Corrigan. Cambridge: Polity Press.

Guedea, Virginia. 1991 *Las Gacetas de México y la medicina: un índice*. México: Universidad Nacional Autónoma de México.

Guerra, Francisco. 1950 *Bibliografia de la materia medica mexicana*. México: La Prensa Medica Mexicana.

——. 1969 "The Role of Religion in Spanish American Medicine." In *Medicine and Culture: proceedings of a historical symposium organized jointly by the Welcome Institute of the History of Medicine, London, and the Wenner-Gren Foundation for Anthropological Research, New York*. Edited by F.N.L. Poynter. London: Welcome Institute of the History of Medicine.

Haines, Michael R. and Richard H. Steckel, editors. 2000 *A Population History of North America*. Cambridge: Cambridge University Press.

Hannaway, Caroline. 1993 "Environment and Miasmata." In *Companion Encyclopedia of the History of Medicine*, vol. 1.Edited by W.F. Bynum and Roy Porter. London: Routledge.

Hernández, Francisco. 1959 *Historia natural de la Nueva España*. 2 vols. México: UNAM.

Hernández Sáenz, Luz María. 1997 *Learning to Heal: The Medical Profession in Colonial Mexico, 1767–1831*. Peter Lang Publishers.

Howard, David A. 1980 *The Royal Indian Hospital of Mexico City*. Temple: Arizona State University, Center for Latin American Studies.

Humboldt, Alexander de. 1973 *Ensayo politico sobre el reino de la Nueva España*. México: Editorial Porrúa, S.A.

Ingham, John M. 1970 "On Mexican Folk Medicine," *American Anthropologist* 72, pp. 76–87.

——. 1986 *Mary, Michael, and Lucifer: Folk Catholicism in Central Mexico*. Austin: University of Texas Press.

Izquierdo, J.Joaquin. 1949 *Raudon, cirujano poblano de 1810: aspectos de la cirugia mexicana de principios del siglo XIX en torno de una vida*. Mexico: Ediciones Ciencia.

Jarcho, Saul. 1957 "Medicine in Sixteenth Century New Spain as Illustrated by the Writings of Bravo, Farfan, and Vargas Machuca." *Bulletin of the History of Medicine*, vol. XXXI, Sept.-Oct. 1957, No.5, PP.425–41.

Jiménez Olivares, Ernestina. 2000 *Los médicos en el Santo Oficio*. México: Departamento de Historia y Filosofía de la Medicina, Facultad de Medicina/UNAM.

Kay, Margarita. 1987 "Lay Theory of Healing in Northwestern New Spain," *Social Science and Medicine*, vol. 24, no.12, pp.1051–1060.

Kelly, Isabel. 1965 *Folk Practices in North Mexico: Birth Customs, Folk Medicine, and Spiritualism in the Laguna Zone*, Austin: University of Texas Press.

Kiple, Kenneth F. 1993 "The Ecology of Disease." In *Companion Enclyclopedia of the History of Medicine*, vol. 1. Edited by W.F. Bynum and Roy Porter. London: Routledge.

Kiple, Kenneth F. and Kriemhild Coneè Ornelas, editors. 2000 *The Cambridge History of Food*. 2 volumes. Cambridge: Cambridge University Press.

Knaut, Andrew L. 1997 "Yellow Fever and the Late Colonial Public Health Response in the Port of Veracruz." *HAHR*, Volume 77, no. 4 (November), pp. 619–644.

Lanning, John Tate. 1969 "The Illict Practice of Medicine in the Spanish Empire of America." In *Homenaje a Don José María de la Peña y Camara*. Madrid: Ediciones José Porrúa Turanzas.

———. 1974 *Pedro de la Torre: Doctor to Conquerors*. Baton Rouge: Louisiana State University Press.

———. 1985 *The Royal Protomedicato*. Durham: Duke University Press.

Lawrence, Ghislaine. 1993 "Surgery (traditional)." In *Companion Enclyclopedia of the History of Medicine*, vol. 2. Edited by W.F. Bynum and Roy Porter. London: Routledge.

Lawrence, Susan. 1993 "Medical Education." In *Companion Enclyclopedia of the History of Medicine*, vol. 2. Edited by W.F. Bynum and Roy Porter. London: Routledge.

Leiby, John S. 1992 "San Hipólito's Treatment of the Mentally Ill in Mexico City, 1589–1650." *The Historian* 54 (1), Spring, pp. 491–98.

León, Nicolás. 1910 *La Obstetricia en México. Notas bibliográficas, étnicas, históricas, documentarias y críticas. De los orígenes históricos has el año* 1910. México: Tip. de la Vda. de F. Diaz de Leon, Sucrs.

———. 1982 "Qué era el Matlazáhuatl y qué el Cocolizli en los tiempos precolombinos y en la época hispana?" in *Ensayos sobre la historia de las epidemias en México*, Florescano Mayer, Enrique and Elsa Malvido Miranda, editors. México: Instituto Méxicano del Seguro Social.

Lobera de Avila. 1952 *Banquete de nobles caballeros*. Madrid: Reimpresiones Bibliograficas.

Lockhart, James. 1992 *The Nahuas After the Conquest: A Social and Cultural History of the Indians of Central Mexico, Sixteenth Through Eighteenth Centuries*, Stanford: Stanford University Press.

———. editor and translator. 1993 *We People Here: Nahuatl Accounts of the Conquest of Mexico*. Berkeley: University of California Press.

López Austin, Alfredo. 1974 "Sahagún's Work and the Medicine of the Ancient Nahuas: Possibilities for Study." In *Sixteenth-Century Mexico: The Work of Sahagún*. Edited by Munro S. Edmonson. Albuqueque: University of New Mexico Press.

——. 1984 "Cosmovisión y salud entre los mexicas." In *Historia general de la medicina en México*. General editor, Fernando Martínez Cortés. Volume I, edited by Alfred López Austin and Carlos Viesca Treviño. México: Universidad Nacional Autónoma de México, Academia Nacional de Medicina.

——. 1988 *The Human Body and Ideology: Concepts of the Ancient Nahuas*. Translated by Thelma Ortiz de Montellano and Bernard Ortiz de Montellano. 2 vols. Salt Lake City: University of Utah Press.

López Austin, Alfredo and Carlos Viesca Treviña, editors. 1984 *Historia general de medicina en México: México antiguo*, Vol. I. Fernando Martínez Cortés, general editor. México: UNAM, Academia Nacional de Medicina.

López, Gregorio. 1708 *Tesoro de medicinas para diversas enfermedades. Añadido, corregido y enmendado*, 3rd Edition. Madrid: Imprenta de Música.

López de Hinojosos, Alonso. 1977 *Suma y recopilacíon de cirugía con un arte para sangrar muy útil y provechosa.* México: Academia Nacional de Medicina.

Loudon, Irvine S.L. 1993 "Childbirth." In *Companion Enclyclopedia of the History of Medicine*, vol. 2. Edited by W.F. Bynum and Roy Porter. London: Routledge.

Maldonado López, Celia. 1995 *Ciudad de México, 1800–1860: epidemias y población*, México: Instituto Nacional de Antropologia e Historia.

Márques Morfin, Lourdes. 1980 *Sociodad colonial y enfermedad: un ensayo de osteopathología diferencial*. México: Instituto Nacional de Antropología.

Márques Morfin, Lourdes and M.E. Peraza, J. Gamboa, T. Miranda. 1982.
Playa del Carmen, una población de la costa oriental en el postclásicoL (un estudio osteológico). México: Instituto Nacional de Antropología Física.

Márques Morfín, Lourdes and Robert McCaa, Rebecca Storey, Andres del Angel. 2002 "Health and Nutrition in Prehispanic Mesoamerica." In *The Backbone of History: Health and Nutrition in the Western Hemisphere*. Edited by Richard H. Steckel and Jerome C. Rose. Cambridge: Cambridge University Press.

McCaa, Robert. 1993 "The Peopling of Nineteenth-Century Mexico: Critical Scrutiny of a Censured Century," *Statistical Abstract of Latin America*. Vol. 30, part 1. Edited by James W. Wilke, Carlos Alberto Contreras, and Christof Anders Weber. Los Angeles: UCLA Latin American Center Publications.

——. 1995 "Spanish and Nahuatl Views on Smallpox and Demographic Catastrophe in Mexico," *Journal of Interdisciplinary History*, vol.XXV:3 (Winter), pp.397–431.

——. 2000 "The Peopling of Mexico from Origins to Revolution," *A Population History of North America*. Edited by Michael R. Haines and Richard H. Steckel. Cambridge: Cambridge University Press.

Mendez, Christobal. 1960 *Book of Bodily Exercise*. Translated by Francisco Guerra, edited by Frederick G. Kilgour. New Haven: Elizabeth Licht.

Mendieta, Fray Gerónimo de. 1945 *Historia eclesiástica indiana*. 4 vols. México: Editorial Salvador Chávez Hayhoe.

Molina del Villar, América. 2001 *La Nueva España y el matlazahuatl, 1736 1739*. México, D.F.: Centro de Investigaciones y Estudios Superiores en Antropolgía Social; y El Colegio de Michoacán, A.C.

Motolinía, Toribio de Benavente. 1971 *Memoriales o Libro de las cosas de la Nueva España y de los naturales de ella*. México: Universidad Nacional Autónoma de México.

Muñuz Garrido, Rafael. 1967 "Empiricos sanitarios españoles de los siglos XVI y XVII," *Cuadernos de historia de medicina española*, vol.6, pp.101–133.

Mureil, Josefina. 1956 *Hospitals de la Nueva España*. 2 vols. México: Publicaciones del Instituto de Historia, no.35.

New World Orders: Casta Painting and Colonial Latin America, 1996, Ilona Katzew, Curator, New York: Americas Society Art Gallery.

Newman, Marshall T. 1976 "Aboriginal New World Epidemiology and Medical Care, and the Impact of Old World Disease Imports," *Physical Anthropology*, November, vol. 45, pp.667–72.

Nutton, Vivian. 1993 "Humoralism." In *Companion Enclyclopedia of the History of Medicine*, vol. 1. Edited by W.F. Bynum and Roy Porter. London: Routledge.

Oktavec, Eileen. 1995 *Answered Prayers: Miracles and Milagros along the Border*. Tucson: University of Arizona Press.

Oriel, J.D. 1994 *The Scars of Venus: A History of Venereology*. London: Springer-Verlag.

Ortiz de Montellano, Bernard R. 1994 *Aztec Medicine, Health, and Nutrition*. New Brunswick, NJ: Rutgers University Press.

Otte, Enrique. 1993 *Cartas Privadas de Emigrantes a Indias, 1540–1616*. México: Fondo de Cultura Económica.

Pagden, Anthony, editor and translator. 1986 *Hernán Cortés: Letters from Mexico*. New Haven: Yale University Press.

Park, Katherine. 1992 "Medicine and Society in Medieval Europe, 500–1500." In *Medicine in Society: Historical Essays*. Editied by Andrew Wear. Cambridge: Cambridge Univeristy Press.

Pelling, Margaret. 1983 "Medicine since 1500." In *Information Sources in the History of Science and Medicine*. Edited by P. Corsi and P. Weindling. London: Butterworth.

——. 1986 "Appearance and Reality: Barber-Surgeons, the Body and Disease." In *London 1500–1700: The Making of the Metropolis*. Edited by A.L. Beier and R. Finaly. New York: Longman.

——. 1998 *The Common Lot: Sickness, Medical Occupations and the Urban Poor in Early Modern England*. London: Longman.

Pelling, Margaret and Charles Webster. 1979 "Medical Practioners." In *Health, Medicine and Mortality in the Sixteenth-Century*. Edited by Charles Webster. Cambridge: Cambridge University Press.

Perdiguero, Enrique. 1992 "The Popularization of Medicine during the Spanish Enlightment." In *The Popularization of Medicine, 1650–1850*. Edited by Roy Porter. London: Routledge.

Pilcher, Jeffery M. 1998 *¡Que vivan los tamales! Food and the Making of Mexican Identity*. Albuqerque: University of New Mexico Press.

Porter, Roy, editor. 1985 *Patients and Practioners: Lay Perceptions of Medicine in Pre-industrial society*. Cambridge: Cambridge University Press.

——. 1985 "The Patient's View: Doing Medical History from Below," *Theory and Society*, 14, pp. 175–198.

——. 1989 *Health for Sale: Quackery in England, 1660–1850*. Manchester: Manchester University Press.

——, editor. 1992 *The Popularization of Medicine, 1650–1850*. London: Routledge.

——. 1997 *The Greatest Benefit to Mankind: A Medical History of Humanity*, New York: W.W. Norton & Company.

Porter, Roy & Dorthy Porter. 1988 *In Sickness and in Health: The British Experience 1650–1850*. London: Fourth Estate.

Porter, Roy, and Andrew Wear, editors. 1987 *Problems and Methods in the History of Medicine*, London: Groom Helm.

Prem, Hanns J. 1991 "Disease Outbreaks in Central Mexico during the Sixteenth Century," in *Secret Judgements of God: Old World Disease in Colonial Spanish America*. Edited by Noble David Cook and W.Geogre Lovell. Norman: University of Oklahoma Press.

Quezada, Noemi. 1989 *Enfermedad y maleficio: el curandero en el México colonial*, México D.F.: Universidad Nacional Autonoma de México.

Quiñones Keber, Eloise. 1995 *Codex Tellerianso-Remensis: Rituals, Divination, and History in a Pictoral Aztec Manuscript*. Austin: Univeristy of Texas Press.

Risse, Gunter B. 1987 "Medicine in New Spain," in *Medicine in the New World: New Spain, New France, and New England*. Edited by Ronald L. Numbers. Knoxville: University of Tennessee Press.

Robinson, David J. 1980 *Research inventory of the Mexican Collection of Colonial Parish Registers*, Salt Lake City: University of Utah Press.

Rodriguez, Martha Eugenia. 2000 *Contaminación e insalubridad en la ciudad de México en el siglo XVIII*. México: Departamento de Historia y Filosofiía de la Medicina, Falcultad de Medicina/UNAM.

Rojo Vega, Anastasio. 1993 *Enfermos y sanadores en la Castilla del siglo XVI*. Valladolid: Universidad de Valladolid.

Rosenberg, Charles E. and Janet Golden, editors. 1992 *Framing Disease: Studies in Cultural History*, New Brunswick: Ruthers University Press.

Ruiz de Alarcón, Hernando. 1984 *Treatise on the Heathen Superstitions That Today Live Among the Indians Native to This New Spain, 1629*. Translated and edited by J.Richard Andrews and Ross Hassig. Norman: University of Oaklahoma Press.

Sahagún, Fray Bernardino de. 1950–69 *Florentine Codex, General History of the Things of New Spain*. 13 vols. Edited and Translated by C.E.Dibble and A.J.O. Anderson. Salt Lake City: University of Utah Press.

——. 1956 *Historia general de las cosas de la Nueva España*. 4 vols. Edited by A.M. Garibay. México: Editorial Porrúa.

Sanchez Lara, Rosa María. 1990 *Los retablos populares: exvotos pintados*. Mexico: Universidad Nacional Autonoma de Mexico y Instituto de Investigaciones Esteticas.

Sanfilippo Borrás, José. 1992 "La atención dental durante el virreinato." In *Temas medicos de la Nueva España*. Edited by Enrique Cárdenas de la Peña. México:Instituto Cultual Domecq, A.C.

Schmidtlein, Adolfo. 1978 *Un médico alemán en el México de Maximiliano: Cartas de Adolfo Schmidtlein a sus padres, 1866–1874*. México: C. Amor S.

Shields, W.J., editor. 1982 *The Church and Healing*. Oxford: Basil Blackwell.

Simmons, Ozzie G. 1969 "Popular and Modern Medicine in Mestizo Communities of Coastal Peru and Chile." In *The Cross-Cultural Approach to Health Behavior*. Edited by L. Riddick Lynch. Rutherford: Farileigh Dickison University Press.

Siraisi, Nancy G. 1990 *Medieval & Early Renaissance Medicine: An Introduction to Knowledge and Practice*, Chicago: University of Chicago Press.

Soldatenko-Gutiérrez, Michael. 1988 *The Mexican Medical Tradition: The Clash of Nahuatl and Spanish Medical Styles. A Bibliography*. Chicano Studies Research Center, UCLA.

Somolinos d'Ardpos, German. 1982 "Las epidemias en México durante el siglo XVI." In *Ensayos sobre la historia de las epidemias en México*. Edited by Enrique Florescano and Elas Malvido Miranda. México: Instituto Mexicano del Seguro Social.

Spink, Wesley W., M.D. 1978 *Infectious Diseases: Prevention and Treatment in the Nineteenth and Twentieth Centuries*. Minneapolis: University of Minnesota Press.

Storey, Rebecca. 1992 *Life and Death in the Ancient City of Teotihuacan: a Modern Paleodemographic Synthesis*. Tuscaloosa:University of Alabama Press.

Taylor, William B. 1979 *Drinking, Homicide, & Rebellion in Colonial Mexican Villages*. Standford: Stanford University Press.

Thomas, Keith V. 1971 *Religion and the Decline of Magic: Studies in Popular Beliefs in Sixteenth and Seventeenth-Century England*, London: Weidenfeld & Nicolson.

Ubelaker, Douglas H. 2000 "Patterns of Disease in Early North American Populations." In *A Population History of North America*. Edited by Michael R. Haines and Richard H. Steckel. Cambridge: Cambridge University Press.

Valdizán, Hermilio and Angel Maldonaldo. 1922 *La medicina popular peruana*. 3 vols. Lima: Imprenta Torres Aguirre.

Varas Machuca, D. Bernardo de. 1892 *Milicia y descripción de Las Indias*. 2 vols. Madrid: Librería de Victoriano Suarez.

Viesca Teviño, Carlos. 1986 *Medicina prehispánica de México. El conocimiento médico de lo nahuas*. México: Panorama Editorial.

——. 1984 "Prevención y terapeúticas mexicas." In *Historia general de la medicina en México*. General editor, Fernando Martínez Cortés. Volume I, edited by Alfred López Austin and Carlos Viesca Treviño. México: Universidad Nacional Autónoma de México, Academia Nacional de Medicina.

——. 1984 "El Médico Mexica." In *Historia general de la medicina en México*. General editor, Fernando Martínez Cortés. Volume I, edited by Alfred López Austin and Carlos Viesca Treviño. México: Universidad Nacional Autónoma de México, Academia Nacional de Medicina.

——. 1982 "Hambruna y epidemia en Anáhuac (1450–1454) en la época de Moctezuma Illhuicamina." In *Ensayos sobre la historia de las epidemias en México*. Edited by Enrique Florescano and Elsa Malvido Miranda. México: Instituto Méxicano del Seguro Social.

Vigarello, Georges. 1988 *Concepts of Cleanliness: Changing Attitudes in France since the Middle Ages*. Translated by Jean Birrell. Cambridge: Cambridge University Press.

Venegas, Juan Manuel, 1788 *Compendio de la medicina práctica en que se declara lacónicamente lo mas útil de ella, que el autor tiene observado en estas regiones de Nueva España, para casi todas las enfermedades que acometen al cuerpo humano*, México: Felipe de Zuñiga y Ontiveros.

Voits, Linda E. and Michael R. McVaugh, editors. 1984 "A Latin Technical Phlebotomy and its Middle English Translation." *Transactions of the American Philosophical Society*, vol. 74, part II.

Wagner, Henry R. 1929 *Spanish Voyages to the Northwest Coast of America in the Sixteenth Century*. San Francisco: California Historical Society.

Ward, James S. 1972 *Yellow Fever in Latin America: A Geographical Study*. London: Center for Latin American Studies-University of Liverpool.

Wear, Andrew. 1993 "The History of Personal Hygiene." In *Companion Encyclopedia of the History of Medicine*, vol. 2. Edited by W.F. Bynum and Roy Porter. London: Routledge.

Weinberger, Margaret J. 2000 "Pica." In *The Cambridge World History of Food*. Vol. 1. Edited by Kenneth F. Kiple and Kriemhild Coneè Ornelas. Cambridge: Cambridge University Press.

Wilson, Adrian. 1985 "Participant or Patient? Seventeenth Century Childbirth from the mother's point of view. In *Patients and Practioners: Lay Perceptions of Medicine in Pre-industrial Society*. Edited by Roy Porter. Cambridge: Cambridge University Press.

Whitmore, Thomas M. 1992 *Disease and Death in Early Colonial Mexico: Simulating Amerindian Depopulation*. Dellplain Latin American Studies, No. 28, Boulder: Westview Press.

Wyngaarden, James B., M.D., Lloyd H. Smith Jr., M.D., and J. Claude Bennett, M.D., Editors. 1992 *Cecil Textbook of Medicine, 19th Edition*. Philadelphia: W.B. Saunders Company.

Zinsser, Hans. 1963 *Rats, Lice and History*. Boston: The Atlantic Monthly Press.

ELECTRONIC RESOURCES

On Mesoamerican Cultures

Ancient Mesoamerican Writing

Aztec Manuscripts: European Paper Manuscripts

Foundation for the Advancement of Mesoamerican Studies, Inc.

Mesoamerican Codices in the University Libraries, University at Albany, State University of New York

Mesoweb: An Exploration of Mesoamerican Cultures
Pre-Columbian Program at Dumbarton Oaks
Prehispanic Calendars

On New Spain, Spanish America

Introduction to the Relaciones Geográficas de América
Latin American Network Information Center: Mexico
Relaciones Geográficas Collection, Benson Latin American Collection, the University of Texas at Austin
Sources and General Resources on Latin America
Vistas: Visual Culture in Spanish America, 1520–1820

On the History of Medicine

History of Medicine, United States National Library of Medicine, National Institutes of Health

GLOSSARY

APOSTEMA apostems or fluid-filled swellings.

BUBAS common name for syphilis in sixteenth century; a catch-all term that described a wide collection of symptoms that involved swellings and sores on different parts of the body.

CALENTURA fever.

CASTAS a generic term for people of mixed race in colonial Spanish America.

CHAPETÓN recently arrived immigrant from Spain.

CHAPETONADA illness that struck recently arrived Spaniards in sixteenth-century Mexico.

COCOLITZLE great plague or illness.

CRIOLLO creole; people of Spanish origin born in Spanish America.

DESTEMPLANZA a disequilibrium in the body's four humors.

DOLOR DE COSTADO "pain in the side." Frequently mentioned disease in colonial period; a group of symptoms common to many diseases, such as pleurisy, emphysema, pneumonia, or tuberculosis.

ESCORBUTO scurvy.

EX-VOTO small votive paintings produced to tell the story of a threatening event from which the subject has been delivered miraculously through the intervention of a divine figure, to whom thanks are reverently offered.

FIEBRE AMARILLA yellow fever.

FLORENTINE CODEX an encyclopedia of Nahua culture and life in precontact Mexico, composed under the auspices of Fray Bernardo de Sahagún during the sixteenth century. Contains images as well as text written in Spanish and Náhuatl.

GENTE DE RAZON "civilized" people.

GUAIACUM wood from a tree native to the West Indies, used as a medicine, especially for syphilis; sometimes called "palo santo."

LIMPIEZA DE SANGRE "purity of blood"; the absence of Jewish or Muslim ancestors. In order to hold privileges, public offices, or enter the university one had to prove their blood purity.

IHIYOTL animistic force residing in the liver; linked to one's passions.

MATLAZÁHUATL epidemic illness, usually associated with typhus.

MORBO GÁLICO the French Disease, or syphilis.

NÁHUATL Uto-Aztecan language spoken by native Mexicans who, in preconquest era, inhabited the central Valley of Mexico and points southeast, as far as Guatemala.

NEYOLMELAHUALIZTLI Nahuas' rite of confession, or "straightening one's heart," a practice that restored internal equilibrium.

OLOLIUHQUI various hallucinogenic plants, among them *Rivea corymbosa*.

PARTERA midwife.

PASMO respiratory illness.

PESTE pestilence.

PINTURA DE CASTAS colonial-era paintings showing different racial mixes of people.

PLETHORA in humoral medicine, the condition of too much blood, resulting in an imbalance of the humors. Usually treated with phlebotomy.

PROTOMEDICATO royal board of officials that regulated the practice of medicine in Spain and its colonies in the Americas.

PROTOMÉDICO chief medical officer.

PULQUE fermented drink made from the juice of maguey plant. Lightly alcoholic.

RELACIONES GEOGRÁFICAS Responses to a questionnaire initiated by the Spanish Crown in 1577 requesting information about Spanish held territories in the Americas. They contain valuable information about indigenous lifestyle and conditions in the sixteenth century. For more information, see http://www.lib.utexas.edu/benson/rg/.

SANGÍAS bleedings.

SUPERFLUITIES buildup of matter in the body, which causes an imbalance in the humors; caused by eating too much, or eating the wrong foods.

TABARDILLO typhus; name is in reference to the characteristic rash that covers the body like a "tabard" or sleeveless cloak.

TEMAZCAL Mesoamerican steam bath; used therapeutically in indigenous medicine.

TEYOLIA (OR **yolia**) animate force residing in the heart; responsible for one's knowledge, emotions, and personality; separated from an individual after death.

TEZCATLIPOCA the Nahuas' major deity; associated with the night, death, sexual transgressions, and discord in general; carries a "smoking mirror." Together with Tlazolteotl, he had the power to cause immorality, punish immoral people, and remove impurities from them as well.

TÍCITL (*plural*, **TITICI**) Náhuatl word for healer, or someone skilled in the art of curing.

TLALOC god of rains; leading member of the Rain-Moisture-Agriculture Fertility Complex.

TLAZOLLI filth, garbage, polluting matter; "matter out of place."

TLAZOLTEOTL "Filth Deity"; goddess of dust and filth, and of persons "tainted" with polluting filth, like adulterers and promiscuous women. Together with Tezcatlipoca, she had the power to cause immorality, punish immoral people, and remove impurities from them as well.

TLAZOLMIQUIZTLI illness caused by someone in a state of filth, usually one who has committed sexual transgressions; literally, "illness of filth."

TONALLI an animate force residing in the head, related to the sun and heat; a day in the 260-day calendar; one's personal destiny due to one's day of birth.

VÓMITO PRIETO (or **NEGRO**) the "black vomit," or yellow fever.

GPSR Authorized Representative: Easy Access System Europe, Mustamäe tee 50, 10621 Tallinn, Estonia, gpsr.requests@easproject.com

www.ingramcontent.com/pod-product-compliance
Ingram Content Group UK Ltd.
Pitfield, Milton Keynes, MK11 3LW, UK
UKHW042338180326
469069UK00006B/1272/J

* 9 7 8 0 2 3 1 1 4 2 4 0 3 *